curly
girl

THE HANDBOOK

curly girl

THE HANDBOOK

EXPANDED SECOND EDITION

by Lorraine Massey

with Michele Bender

Photographs by Gabrielle Revere

WORKMAN PUBLISHING COMPANY • NEW YORK

Library of Congress Cataloging-in-Publication Data is available.

ISBN 978-0-7611-5678-9

Design by Lidija Tomas
Cover design by Janet Vicario
Workman books are available at special discounts when purchased in bulk for premiums and sales promotions as well as for fund-raising or educational use. Special editions or book excerpts can also be created to specification. For details, contact the Special Sales Director at the address below or send an e-mail to specialmarkets@workman.com.

Workman Publishing Company, Inc.
225 Varick Street
New York, NY 10014-4381
www.workman.com

Printed in China
First printing December 2010
10 9 8 7 6 5 4

Photography Credits:

COVER PHOTOGRAPHY by GABRIELLE REVERE (Front and Back)

Author photo Courtesy of Lorraine Massey

ORIGINAL PHOTOGRAPHY BY GABRIELLE REVERE: vi top, vii top and middle, 1 (all images), 7, 9, 18, 21 left, 22 left, 23 left, 24 left, 25 left, 26 left, 27 left, 32, 33, 37 left and right, 38–41 (all images), 42 right, 44–47 (all images), 48 left, 50–61 (all images), 66 top and bottom, 67 top left, 67 top and bottom right, 68 left, 70, 71, 75, 77, 90–93 (all images), 94 right, 96–99 (all images), 102–104 (all images), 106–110 (all images), 112–116 (all images), 118, 121 right, 123 bottom, 124–126 (all images), 134–137 (all images), 138 top, 140 right, 151 right, 156, 159–161 (all images), 162 left middle and bottom, 162 right top and bottom, 163–164 (all images), 165 top left and right, 167 (all images), 170 (all images), 172 (all images).

ADDITIONAL PHOTOGRAPHY:

AGE FOTOSTOCK: Beauty Photo Studio, 171 left; Lucenet Patrice, 6; ASSOCIATED PRESS: 27 right; ERIC BROWN: vi bottom, vii bottom, viii, x (all images), 5 bottom, 13 top, 19, 20, 21 center, 22 center, 23 center, 24 center, 25 center, 26 center, 27 center, 29, 36 bottom right, 38, 67 bottom left, 94 left, 101, 157, 162 top left, 165 bottom left, 171 right; FOTOLIA: Monika Adamczyk, 87; Africa, 88; Barbro Bergfeldt, 84 top; Richardo Bhering, 128 left; Norman Chan, 86; cs333, 36 left; Philip Date, 151 left; EastWest Imaging, 149; Ewa Brozek, 132; eyewave, 84 bottom; Daniel Hughes, 82; kalou1927, 152; Kurhan, 144; Marylooo, 35 top; MM, 73; Oleg Shelomentsev, 119; Jason Stitt, 147 right; vlad valentina, 42 left, 83; volff, 85; Elliot Westacott, 154; ZTS, 35 bottom; PHOTOFEST: 30; PHOTO RESEARCHERS: Biophoto Associates, 15 right; John Durham/Science Photo Library, 15 left; Oliver Meckes, 11; RETNA: 22 left.

COURTESY PHOTOS:

Michele Bender, 76; Robin Berger, 78 left and right; Elizabeth Cantor, 174 bottom; Debrah Chiel, 10 left and right; Karen Ferleger, 17 left and right; Sandra Gering, 117 left and right; Michael Graeser, 138 bottom left and right; Clifton and Miriam Green, 133 left and right; Benjamin Griffiths, 175 left and right; David Lopez, 28, 128, 142, 143, 147 bottom left, 148, 150 left and right, 173; Christine Carter Lynch, 69 left and right; Lorraine Massey, v, xiii, 2, 3, 4, 5 top, 16, 48 left, 72, 122, 123 top and middle, 140 (3 images on left), 145 top and bottom, 146 top and bottom, 153, 181 top and bottom, 188 (all images); Denise McCoy, 111 (all images); Jo Newman, 49 left and right; Shelly Ozkan, 31, 130; Patti Page, 89 left and right; Elizabeth Pilar, 43 left and right; Jordan Pacitti, 139, 174 top; Sophie Portnoy, 131; Netta Rabin, 105; Jesse Reese, 8 left and right; Allen Salkin, 141; Asa and Clara Schiller, 129 left and right; Noelle Smith, 178 left and right; Stephanie Trusty, 62 left and right; Vickie Vela, 176 bottom; Vida, 63, 64 (all images); Claire Warren, 168; Nathalie Wechsler, 121 left; Julie Weiss 81.

ILLUSTRATION:

Robert Risko; used with permission of the *Chicago Tribune* 166.

To my mother,
Jemima Rutherford Bathgate Massey Dance

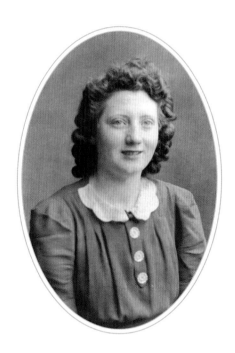

and to Kaih, Shey, Dylan, Veronica, and Venaih

contents

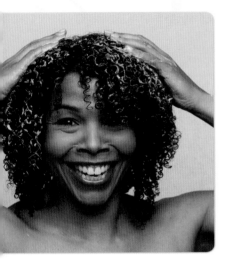

A pre-cleanse treatment to hydrate the hair, page 66

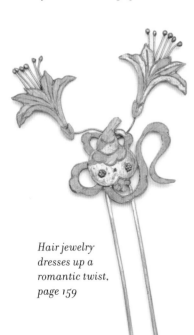

Hair jewelry dresses up a romantic twist, page 159

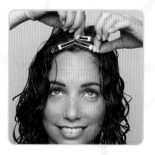

The clipping technique, page 41

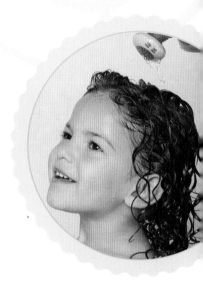

Teaching kids to love their curls, page 128

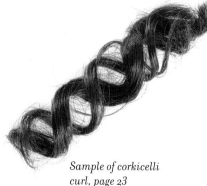

Sample of corkicelli curl, page 23

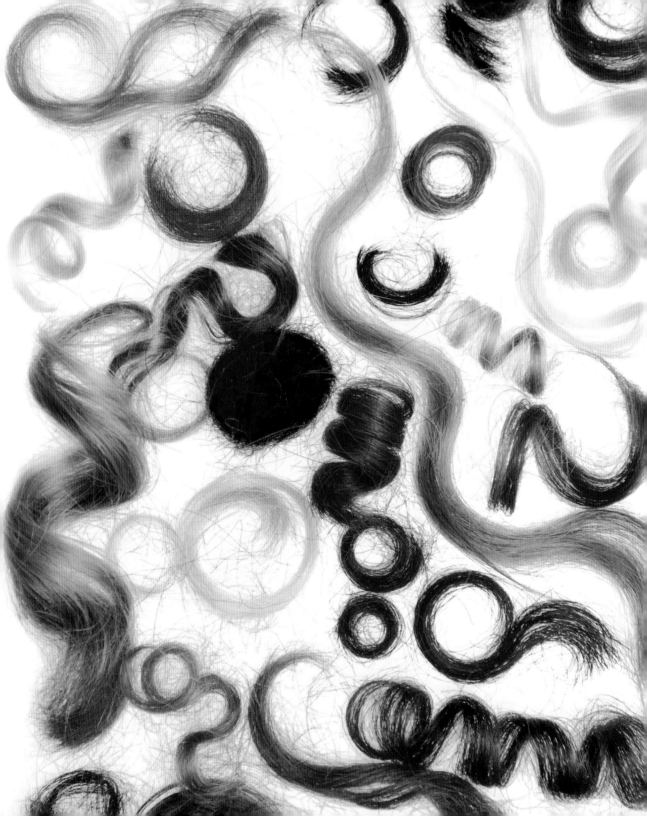

introduction

LOCKS TO TALK ABOUT

A lot has changed in the world of curls since the first version of *Curly Girl* came out ten years ago. For so many years, ringlets, corkscrews, and waves were the ugly ducklings of the hair world, viewed as a symptom to be treated, an aberration to be tamed, rather than a part of nature. When you'd go to the hairdresser, there was an "obviously, you don't want those curls" attitude and an expectation that you should be grateful to your stylist for blow-drying your hair straight after a cut. In fact, at a recent hair convention, a hairdresser came over to me and said, "If you let me blow-dry your hair, you'll fall in love with me." (Hardly!)

Straighten your hair, and you might be happy for a day. Learn to love and care for your curls, and you'll be happy for life!

Despite the strides many curly girls have made to accept and understand their curls, the hairdresser's comment is typical of the hair community's mentality and evidence that straight hair still rules. Here are some revealing facts and stats: Flat irons are the top-selling item in the hair care industry. At one point, a transatlantic airline offered these appliances to passengers so they could straighten their strands before landing (while the rest of us in the plane had to endure the smell of burning hair). The number one service in salons worldwide is blow-drying (which I call blow-*frying* because of its damage to your hair), and an amazing $9 billion–plus worth of hair-straightening products are sold annually. Recently a well-known hair product company boasted about creating a pill that claims to change your DNA to straighten your curls. (Can't you just imagine the future news story: "Woman has symptoms of paralysis, temporary blindness, and slurred speech, but she's happy that her hair is finally straight!")

For the past ten years, I've spent my days with hundreds of loyal clients as well as the 30,000 new clients who come to our Devachan Salons each year, many traveling long distances to experience the curly transformation firsthand. We listen to their concerns and study their curls. I'm fascinated by the amazing beauty and diversity of natural curls and have started a collection of samples, some of which are shown, right. Yet there is still many a curly girl hiding beneath blown-out, straightened, flattened strands. And there are still many questions about curly hair that need answers.

Readers have asked me about things that weren't in the first version of *Curly Girl*—like how to trim their own hair, how to make their waves behave, what products to use, and how to grow out their chemically straightened strands to go back

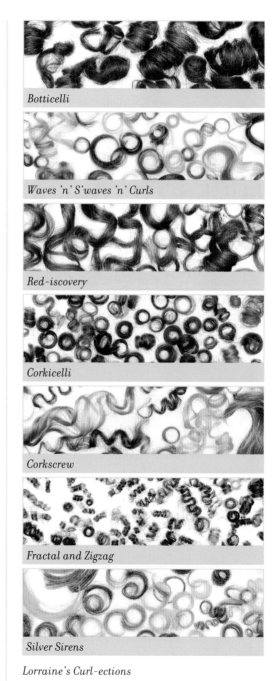

Botticelli

Waves 'n' S'waves 'n' Curls

Red-iscovery

Corkicelli

Corkscrew

Fractal and Zigzag

Silver Sirens

Lorraine's Curl-ections

to their curly roots—so I address those issues in this book. In the last decade, I've also watched some of my wonderful client friends bravely go through cancer treatments, so I've added a section on chemo curls.

The other thing that's happened since I wrote the first book is the birth of the DevaCurl line of products. Early on, my partner Denis DaSilva and I tried various product lines at our salon, but we couldn't find any that helped curly hair look its best. We also experimented with whipping up our own homemade formulas (like a lavender spray, which later developed into DevaCurl Mist-er Right, and a sulfate-free cleanser, called No-Poo) because detergents are especially damaging to curly hair. But our clients were begging for these products that weren't on the market. So we began interviewing dozens of chemists and finally found one who was open to formulating products that were good for the hair. Over the course of a year, he created samples that we tested in the salon and sent home with clients. After much tweaking back in the lab, we proudly launched the DevaCurl line of botanical products that is becoming vital in the curly world.

This and so much that I've learned since the first book are on the pages that follow. Plus you get a DVD showing various daily routines for different types of curls, self-trimming, clipping techniques, and curly updos. If you are new to the world of *Curly Girl*, welcome! The book and DVD will teach you a whole new way of living with your curls. Follow the program for your particular type of curls and your hair will be transformed. If you're already a curly girl, it will provide the latest information on how to continue to treat your curls and new ways to love them. Yes, curls have a will of their own, subject to weather and mood, but once you come to accept this, and work *with* your curls instead of against them, they will respond.

It might sound a bit obsessive, but ever since I can remember, my curls have informed and guided my philosophy of living: Every day is a new day and you've got to just go with the flow. Accepting yourself as you are and letting go of what society says you should be are first steps toward freeing yourself. "Free your hair and the rest will follow" became my manifesto. Curls are the wave of the future and this, my curly friends, is just the beginning.

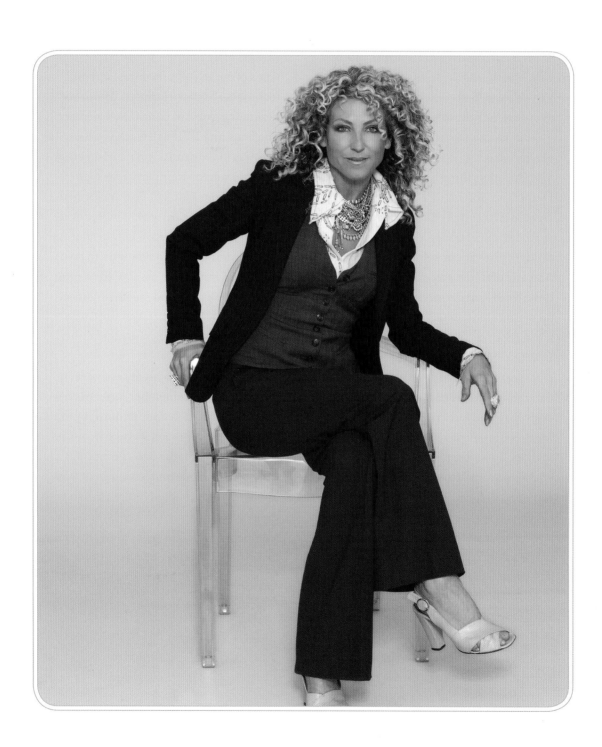

CHAPTER 1

girl meets curl

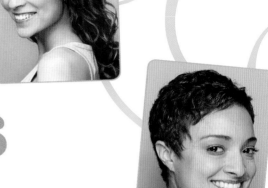

It's your head, not your hair, that needs straightening.

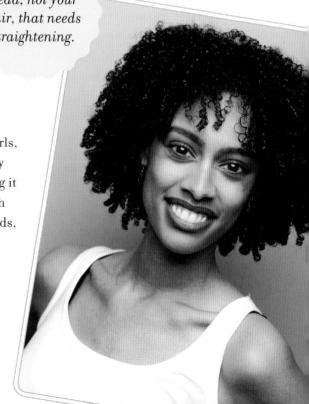

Chances are, if you picked up this book, you belong to the sisterhood of curly girls, women who've been fighting their curly hair for most of their lives, blow-drying it straight, hiding it under hats, pulling it back with rubber bands, disguising it with weaves and braids, or flattening it with anything they could find. Depending on what era you were born into, you may have tried chemical straighteners, blow-fryers (as I call them), flat irons, or gigantic juice-can rollers to straighten your hair. I know all about this.

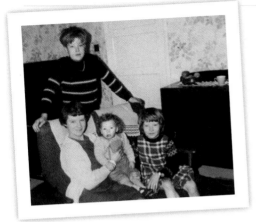

My brothers and sisters made fun of my hair.

Where I was born, in Leicester, England, curly hair was made fun of more than it was accepted. I hated my hair from the moment I was able to look in the mirror and see that, unlike my six brothers and sisters, whose hair seemed appropriately lank, I had corkscrew curls that stuck out all over my head, making me look like Little Orphan Annie. For years I was sure that there'd been some mistake at the hospital and I'd been sent home with the wrong set of parents. For my third birthday, I asked my mother for a straight-haired wig and a grass skirt so I could pretend I was a Polynesian hula dancer. It was a strange request from a toddler living in a poor factory town in the British West Midlands. By the time I was four, I was watching rock stars and actresses on TV swinging their long, stick-straight hair back and forth. If only my hair could swing, I'd think. I'd pull my sweater halfway over my head so that it hung down across my back. Look, I have straight hair, too.

I now realize that I wasn't alone. In this book, you'll find the personal stories of a world of other curly girls who went through the same denial and hair despair I did. We all worried about humid days, when despite all our efforts, our hair would frizz up. We were teased by kids in school ("Hey, Brillo, where'd you get that hair?" or "Sit in the back of the class. I can't see the blackboard through your hair!"), and made to feel that curly hair and therefore, we were inferior.

As I got older, I developed a victim mentality about my curls, thinking that they were a perverse joke played on me by a whimsical universe, a genetic mistake that the gods of beauty had planted in my DNA. I'd spend all day thinking up ways to make my hair stay flat and frizz-free. In my mind, the equation was simple: Straight was beautiful, curly was ugly. A sociologist might point out that for many people, this preference for straight hair was a subtle form of racism. Most of us have been influenced by stereotypes of beauty promoted in the last half of the twentieth century—the white Anglo-Saxon look, with straight blond hair and a pale complexion. Children could have curls— if they were golden—but they'd damn well better straighten out by the time they grew up. I would go to bed at night, my hair tightly wound—imprisoned, actually—around gigantic rollers. (Even at sleepovers!) I'd lie very still lest one should slip off and the curls spring cruelly and sadistically back to life.

So it was inevitable that I decided to become a hairdresser. I'd spent so much time fixing my own hair that I might as well try to make a living fixing others'. I served three years as an apprentice in England, then moved to Hong Kong for four years and became fascinated with my customers' straight hair. Next, I lived in Japan, where the first word of Japanese I learned, of course, was *masuga*, which means "straight." I was surprised to find some curly girls in Japan! (Where do you think Japanese hair straightening comes from?) Even when a few popular TV shows and their gorgeous female stars made long, wavy hair fashionable, I kept mine short. One time a hairdresser gave me a cropped cut called a tunnel cut (see page 100), but despite its length my hair still appeared voluminous. That night I went to a party, and a boy I fancied took one look at me and said, "Your hair looks like a baboon's backside."

That was it! Like an addict who's bottomed out, I realized I couldn't fight my curls anymore. I started letting my hair grow. I stopped blow-frying it. As my curls grew, they turned into spirals, then ringlets. Meanwhile, I tried to find any scrap of information I could about curly hair, but there was nothing available on the subject of curls. All the hair schools I interviewed said, "Hair is hair. We treat curly the same as straight." No wonder so many hairdressers continue to straighten everyone out. I found few curly hair role models, something I realized that I'd been searching for ever since I was five years old. (Back then, I dreamed a fairy curlmother would stop me on the street and say, "Listen to me. I know exactly what to do with your curls." Of course, it never happened.)

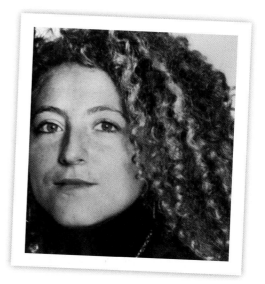

My curls in Hong Kong's 100 percent humidity.

I began conditioning my hair regularly, experimenting with different products, upping the amount of conditioner. I let my hair grow so the soft S's that are my hair's natural shape had room to develop. Eventually my scalp sprouted ringlets, then lengthened into thick corkscrews that spiraled down my shoulders. This was my hair destiny—nature finally taking its course. Recently, a fifty-four-year-old client Miriam was told by a friend, "Finally, you have the hair you were always meant to have!" That is exactly how I felt.

I became totally politicized about curly hair. I saw it almost like an arranged marriage—something I might not have chosen for myself at first, but mine "till death do us part." (In fact, my will forbids anyone to straighten my hair upon my death and contains instructions to the person handling my curls for my funeral.) I vowed that no one was going to straighten my hair or my mind again.

Unfortunately, while I had changed, the world around me hadn't. Straight hair was still the gold standard, especially in Beverly Hills, where I'd gotten a job in a fashionable salon. I had been working there for about a week when the salon owner returned from vacation, meeting me for the first time. He pointed at me, the new girl with politically incorrect curls, and went ballistic. "Someone blow-dry that girl's hair now!" he shouted. Moments later, I left my post at the shampoo bowl and walked. I never looked back.

I moved to New York City, where, for the first time in the life of my curls, I was surrounded by multi-curl-tural people. Jewish, Italian, Latino, and African American people living around me had curly hair that looked like mine! I no longer looked or felt like an outsider.

My friends jokingly accuse me of living in a "curl-centric" world. That may be true, but it's also true that we still live in a world where the straight-hair stereotype has a tremendous hold on our imaginations. Perhaps that explains why so many of us are still in curl denial, why cosmetology schools still teach stylists to cut curls with a flattened, forced, one-dimensional straightness, and why so many

The Beverly Hills salon where my curls were seen as "politically incorrect."

hairdressers are intimidated by curly hair. Rather than working with hair's natural curl and texture, hairdressers have been trained to blow it straight, which takes at least 30 minutes to do (and about 20 seconds to undo if it's humid or raining).

An estimated 65 percent (possibly more) of women have curly or wavy hair. (Take the quiz on page 6 to see if you are one of them.) But too many of us are still at a loss about how to properly care for our hair or, worse, are pretending we have straight hair and mistreating our natural curls. Curly girls need to surrender their weapons of mass hair destruction, like blow-fryers, flat irons, detergent-filled shampoos, straighteners, and weaves. I'm trying to help you and curly girls everywhere with this book, through hairdressing seminars on how to cut curly hair, and in my work as the co-owner of the Devachan Salons and Deva Spa. There, we encourage our clients to accept their hair, love what they have and make the most of it. In other words, to straighten out their heads instead of their hair. After all those years of struggling and being challenged by what I viewed as unruly hair, I have learned that curls are worth fighting for.

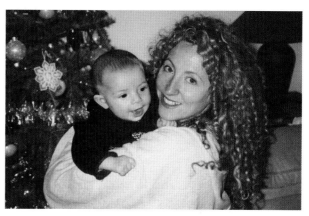

Shey, my future curly girl.

I'm hoping that this book can change the way you approach your curly hair. In it you'll find a complete guide to curls, their origins, their potential, and their needs. You'll learn a radical and logi-curl way to care for your specific curl type and nurture its intrinsic shape. How to cleanse, condition, and style your hair, and how to have it cut respectfully instead of having it sliced, carved, and butchered. You'll wear your curls with pride every day. I promise. It will change your life. So curl up (sorry) and start reading.

Curly Q's

Are you still hiding the truth from the world, maybe even from yourself? Take this simple question-hair to determine whether you're a member of the curly clan.

1. Do you live in fear of humidity, sweating, spontaneous sex, a shower with your lover—or any weather or activity that might unmask you as a curly girl?

2. Do you have your hair professionally blow-dried and then don't wash it for a week (and use powder or dry shampoo that dulls the hair)?

3. Do you find yourself upset (even close to tears) after every haircut?

4. Does your hair develop unwanted volume in humid, hot, or wet weather?

5. Does your budget for products and appliances to fight frizz, straighten, or relax your hair exceed your annual tax-deductible contributions to charity?

6. Are you almost always unhappy with the way your hair looks?

7. Do you worry about your hair before any big occasion, like a wedding or an important business meeting?

8. Do you almost always have a halo of frizz around your head?

9. Do you blow-dry your hair so often that its texture is dry and brittle and there are broken bits of hair on top and in your bangs?

10. Do you often wear your hair tied back so tight that you get a headache?

11. Do your curls make you feel out of control?

12. Look at old photographs and recall how you felt about your hair—and yourself—on the day each picture was taken (if you even have pictures of your bad hair days). Was there a strong correlation between your hair and your mood?

If you answered yes to one or more questions, congratulations! You're a curly girl waiting to happen. Your hair is bristling with movement, longing to break free, waves aching to curl, frizz begging for direction. Read on!

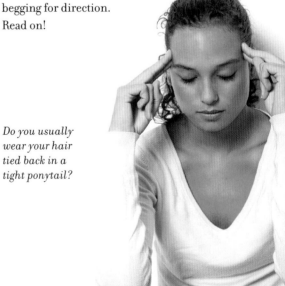

Do you usually wear your hair tied back in a tight ponytail?

ARE YOU A CURLY GIRL?

The Curly 10

I could give you a million compelling reasons to go curly! But let's start with ten:

1. You become freer with your hair. (And you feel more free to be yourself.)

2. Curls make you look younger.

3. Going curly means going green. The detergents (sulfates) in shampoo pollute the water, so living a sulfate-free life helps keep the earth's water supply clean. Not using blow-dryers and flat irons means you're saving electricity.

4. Life is simpler because you don't need any plug-ins for hair care.

5. Curls equal less stress. Your life no longer revolves around the weather.

6. Travel becomes easy. You'll pack fewer products and no appliances, and won't worry about how a new climate will affect your hair.

7. You are more active. You no longer have to skip a dip in the pool or a sweaty workout.

8. If it rains on a special occasion, you won't have to worry.

9. You'll save the time and money you spent on hair appointments.

10. Learning to accept and love your curls means learning to accept and love yourself!

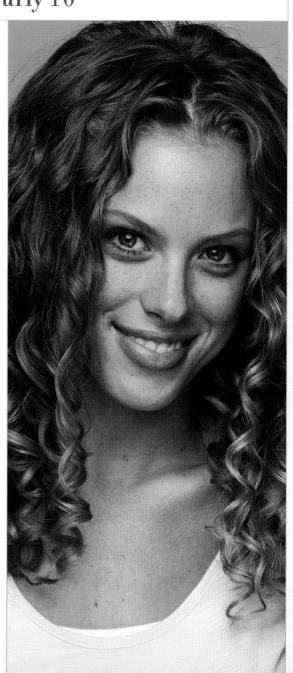

curl confession

Jesse Reese *human resources generalist*

For most of my life I wanted to be like all the girls whose straight-haired ponytails swooshed from side to side. But my curls were simply uninspired. I wore them in a ponytail day in and day out in an attempt to hide the fact that my hair was different. Then in college, I discovered products for curly hair and a salon that knew how to cut my curls and make them look shiny, healthy, and full of life. I had never been more excited to be a curly girl.

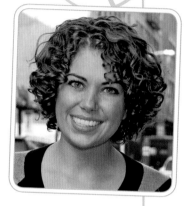

In my senior year, I participated in a mock interview with my university's career center to prepare myself for my upcoming job search. Afterward, the man conducting the faux interview gave me some "constructive" criticism—not about my answers or resume, but about my appearance. "For your real interviews, straighten your hair," he said. "Curly hair is unprofessional." I've never been more offended in my life. I told him that my hair is a part of who I am and I would never work for an employer who wouldn't hire someone because of the shape of her hair.

Loving my curls has changed my outlook on life and helped me become an independent woman. And it has given me the confidence to stand up to people who believe that women must fit a certain mold—a mold that requires straight hair. I am determined to break that mold and show others that curly girls are empowered women and that we are here to stay. We're girls! We have curls! Get used to it!

CHAPTER 2

hair, the inside story

On every curly-haired baby's head, there should be a care label reading: Delicate. No harsh shampoos. No machine drying. Air-dry only. Never iron.

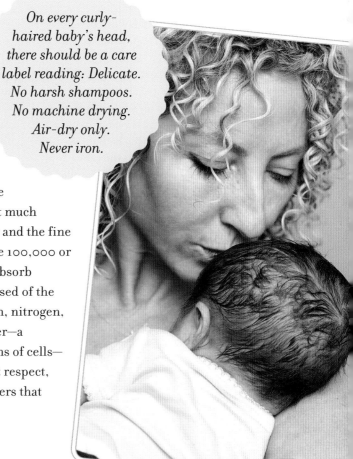

I love care labels in clothes. They make me respect a fabric and think carefully about how I treat it. If only our hair came with a care label! The truth is, there isn't much difference chemically between your hair and the fine wool that comes off a pashmina goat. The 100,000 or so hair fibers on your head stretch and absorb moisture, just like wool, which is composed of the same elements as hair: carbon, hydrogen, nitrogen, oxygen, and sulfur. Because hair is a fiber—a delicate, special fiber made up of millions of cells— it makes sense to treat it with the utmost respect, the way you would the other precious fibers that you own or admire.

curl confession

Deborah Chiel *writer*

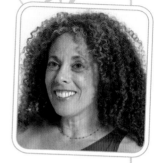

The morning of my father's funeral, I had a really bad hair day. I don't mean to sound disrespectful, but this was my worst nightmare come true. All my life, I'd suffered because of my curly hair: bad cuts, ill-fated attempts to grow my hair long, hours spent straightening it with hideous-smelling chemicals, dates gone bad because my hair had morphed into a giant ball of frizz.

Decades later, I still believe I would've had a more successful high school social life if the sun had been shining and the humidity low as I walked into my first class in a new school. Worst of all were the Saturday mornings of my adolescence, most of which I spent in synagogue because my father was the rabbi. I would stand in front of the mirror, wailing because my hair had taken on shapes not known in nature. But my father refused to accept the frizz factor as a reason not to show up at services. I sat in synagogue week after week, hating my hair, myself, my life. I didn't have a bad hair day. I had a bad hair decade.

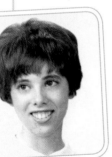

After college, I started therapy, and rehashed how much misery my hair had caused me during my curl-hood, especially as a teenager. My therapist seemed to think that my unhappiness was related to other, more profound issues, but what did she know? Her hair was stick straight.

Years passed. I had my ears pierced, exchanged my glasses for contact lenses, and began to emerge from my curl-related shell. Then came my father's unexpected death from a heart attack. On this most painful occasion of my life, when hundreds of people were expected to attend the funeral, my hair betrayed me. No doubt much of my reaction was displaced grief, but my anti-curl emotions ran deep and had a powerful hold over my psyche.

My story has a happy ending. I eventually met Lorraine, who encouraged me to stop fighting with my hair and cultivate my curls by growing them long. These days, I feel sexier, freer, more flirtatious, even drawn to glitter and sequins. I am constantly astonished and gratified by my curls and people's reactions to them.

You'd never dream of washing a good wool or cashmere sweater with just any old detergent. But most people don't think twice about applying shampoo to the priceless fiber that's sitting on top of their head. The problem is that shampoos have a dirty little secret: They contain harsh detergents such as sodium lauryl sulfate, ammonium laureth sulfate, or sodium laureth sulfate, which are foaming agents found in dishwashing liquid and laundry detergent. Sure, they're good for pots and pans because they cut grease so effectively.

Your hair, on the other hand, needs to retain its natural oils to protect it and your scalp. Stripping them away deprives the hair of necessary moisture, amino acids, and antibodies, and makes it look dry, dull, and lifeless. It also does the same thing to skin. When I was a junior hair assistant in Leicester, England, I'd wash ten to fifteen heads of hair a day and my hands would be chapped and bleeding because of all the detergents in the shampoos. That's not surprising since chemists all over the world have proven that detergents are skin and eye irritants. Still, companies continue to use detergents in shampoos, which were first commercially available after World War II, because they are cheap. And because we're addicted to suds!

You don't have to take my word for it. To see what detergent does to your hair, try this simple experiment in your kitchen: Pour a bit of dishwashing detergent onto a damp sponge and squeeze gently. Voilà, bubbles! Now, hold the sponge under running water and notice that it seems to take forever to rinse it free of the lather. I've done this experiment with various shampoos and soaps and have been shocked to find that in some cases the bubbles were there ten hours later! The point is that you never really get rid of all that detergent. It stays in your hair, and it pollutes our water system.

Shampoo isn't good for any hair, but for curly girls it's a disaster. That's because curly hair is so porous that it absorbs detergent like a sponge. Put it in your hair and it doesn't rinse out. The truth is that lathers don't really cleanse at all. Manufacturers put lathering agents into products so you'll buy into the joy-of-suds myth. You know, those women in TV commercials moaning in ecstasy as they lather up their heads in the shower, then reappear seconds later sporting wonderfully styled hair, shining with vitality. Well, forget the advertising campaigns that put sudsiness right up there next to cleanliness, godliness, and sexiness. It doesn't work that way—

especially for curls—and you don't have to buy into it.

I can't say this too often: *You do not need to use shampoo.* I'm not saying leave your hair dirty. You still must cleanse the hair and scalp, but as you read on, you'll see that I recommend doing so with a sulfate-free cleanser or a botanical conditioner (derived from real plant extracts). You need to give up your lather habit and shampoo dependency. I did and it worked! In the bad old days, I would subject my scalp and hair to a vigorous lathering several times a week, for no good reason except force of habit.

Afterward, for the first two days, my hair would appear to float in space like a helium balloon, defying the laws of gravity and reaching to the heavens above. I had ruffled the surface cuticle and dehydrated the curls. As a result, the cuticle was following its natural instinct—to reach out for moisture from the atmosphere, hence the frizz. Another three days would go by before my hair had recovered enough from the trauma that I was ready to admit we were related. Then we'd happily coexist for the rest of the week (two days), until it was time—according to my self-imposed schedule—for my next shampoo. And the vicious cycle would begin all over again.

I unquestioningly followed this routine, because I'd never found any care instructions that addressed the specific needs of curly, as opposed to straight, hair. Then one morning I looked in the mirror and I had to admit that my hair looked frizz-free and curlicious. According to my schedule, I was due for a shampoo, but I couldn't bear to mess with success. I dared myself to wait another day. One day stretched into a second, then a third, until I'd managed to hold out for almost three weeks. All I did was cleanse my scalp with a spritz of lavender and squeeze some watered-down conditioner onto my hair and scrunch. My hair had never looked better, so I decided to try an experiment: I would see how long I could refrain from washing my hair with detergent-laden shampoo and replace it with what I now call "no-poo." And you know what? The moment I stopped using

HarD WaTer anD CurLy Hair

Hard water contains dissolved salts of calcium and magnesium. When these combine with the sulfates in shampoo, a chemical reaction occurs that makes it even harder to rinse the detergent out and leaves your hair even drier. But it's not all bad news: If you use sulfate-free hair products in areas with hard water, their lack of detergents makes these cleaners even easier to rinse out.

shampoo was the moment I started loving my hair!

Now I live in what I call a no-poo household. I don't use shampoo or detergents at all anymore, not even a drop. I work up a sweat running most mornings in all different environments and I swim in the ocean and pools not far from my home, and yet my scalp smells fresh and my hair has never looked better.

THE CUTICLE IS CRITICAL

If you examine a cross-section of a hair fiber under a microscope, you'll see that it looks like a piece of spaghetti. Growing around the shaft are tiny scales, which cover the cortex or center of the hair like tiles on a roof. Those overlapping tiles are called the cuticle of the hair, and they're essential in protecting each strand and making your hair look good. When the tiles lie flat, they reflect light and your hair shines. When they're ruffled, your hair won't shine because light needs to be reflected off a smooth surface. Detergents, heat from a blow-dryer or flat iron, chemicals, and brushes damage hair by making the cuticle rough and scaly. Instead of lying flat, pieces of cuticle stick

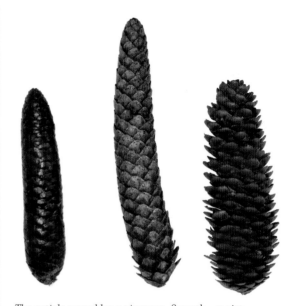

The cuticle resembles a pinecone. Smooth = moist cuticle. Open = dry, frizzed cuticle.

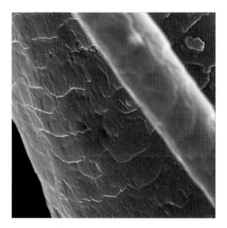

A strand of healthy, well-conditioned hair: The tilelike cuticle lies flat.

out and lock together like Velcro, causing knots, snarls, and tangles.

WHY CURLY HAIR IS DRIER

Most of us treat our hair and scalp as a single entity. But the scalp is very different from the hair. The scalp is skin that needs to be treated the way we treat our facial skin—by cleansing it gently and keeping it moisturized. The hair is a skin appendage made up mainly of a protein called keratin that has a fiberlike consistency. Each hair follicle that produces the hair on our heads is also home to sebaceous (oil) glands, which release sebum, an oily substance that lubricates the hair. One reason experts say curly hair is so much drier than other types of hair is because there are only about 100,000 hairs on a head of curly hair, as opposed to about 120,000 hairs on a head of straight hair. And because there is less curly hair, there are fewer follicles, and therefore fewer sebaceous glands to produce oil. If you have tightly curled hair, the sebum sometimes has trouble getting to the ends, which tend to be especially dry, so you have to compensate with extra moisturizers.

It's possible to have dry hair and an oily scalp. Having combination skin, oily in the T-zone (the chin, nose, and forehead) but dry everywhere else, is one clue that you might have an oily scalp. The sebum and sweat that your scalp produces are sterile and clean but they attract dirt and bacteria, which must be rinsed off regularly to keep the scalp healthy. But it's not necessary to remove all the oils from your scalp; in fact, it's not good for you.

strand of curly hair looks elliptical, with a slight curve in the middle (like ribbon candy). The center indentation makes the hair flex and spiral—in other words, curl. A strand of fractal or zigzag curls is flatter still than a strand of corkscrew curls and has the finest texture, therefore making it the curliest. Wavy hair looks oval under a microscope. Its spiral is gentler and it bends very slightly.

As a rule, curly hair is very fine and straight hair is thicker. Someone with

You need a fine layer of sebum—called the acid mantle—to protect the scalp. My solution is to a give the scalp a firm massage and a good water rinsing followed by conditioner or to spritz the scalp with lavender mist. (See page 83.)

IT'S IN THE GENES

Genetics determine whether your hair is naturally curly or straight. Look at a cross-section of very straight hair and you'll see that its shape is round. (Think of toothpaste coming out of a tube.) A

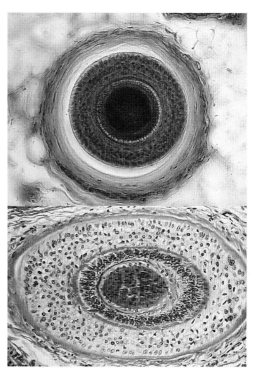

The fiber of straight hair (top) is round; a strand of wavy hair (bottom) is oval.

tight, curly hair may appear to have thick hair because it has such volume, but that's an optical illusion. The curls' spherical shape fills in space and creates the impression of thickness. But each strand is usually baby-fine.

FrIZZ-ASSIST

The main reason we curly girls are not happy with our hair is because of that curly girl nemesis: frizz (which I now call "halo"). In fact, many women don't even know they have gorgeous curls because their hair is suffocating under layers of dreadful, dry frizz. I have become what I call a "frizz-assist" so I can help you understand the science behind frizz. Once you do, you'll never look at it the same way again.

So here's your frizz education: Most of us spend days, months, and years dehydrating our already dry hair with harsh, detergent-filled shampoos, blow-dryers, and chemical treatments. It's the natural inclination of the little strands of your hair to literally lift up off your head and outward to quench their thirst from moisture in the air due to their molecular structure. These lifted hair fibers create a poof of frizz. This is why curly girls who straighten their hair dread days when it's humid or it rains. (I actually have a chart from the 1500s that used hair as a weather barometer! It sounds crazy but it makes sense.)

The solution, however, is simple: moisture. Once the hair fibers are sufficiently hydrated with conditioner, they will hold onto the moisture they need and the frizz will go away. Curly hair is porous, but the conditioner fills the holes a bit like spackle on walls and smoothes the surface. And thanks to gravity, the weight of the conditioner pulls the hair down and even makes it appear longer in some cases. With enough hydration, anyone and everyone can have beautifully defined curls without the frizz!

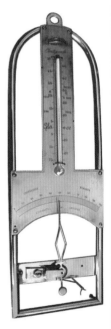

An eighteenth-century hygrometer that used hair to measure humidity.

curl confession

Karen Ferleger *stay-at-home mom*

What was it like growing up with curly hair? In one word: HELL! I looked like Little Orphan Annie until the age of fourteen, when my hair was cut off completely—practically shaved on the sides and back, with little curls on top.

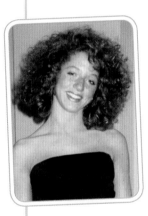

When I was a freshman in college, I was growing my hair out and waiting for my curls to fall. My then-boyfriend's friends called me Ronald McDonald and wanted to know how he could date a person with that hair. (We are now married.)

One of my worst curly hair experiences was when I was a sophomore in college and going to a fraternity formal dance. My hair had finally grown to a little below my ears. I wanted straight hair for the formal, so I went to a salon at a very fancy hotel, where instead of straight hair, I got the puffiest hairdo ever. I was miserable the entire night.

When I moved to New York City after college, I would get my hair blown out once a year on a cold winter day with only good weather predicted. It would take two hours and the hairline around my face would be burnt from the straightener. To top it off, it would only last a day or two—not worth the pain!

After spending literally thousands of dollars on hair products, I found something that worked, and finally learned to love my curls. Still, I do have a monthly nightmare that I am in a salon chair and the stylist cuts off all of my hair again like when I was a kid. I wake up in a panic and quickly reach for my hair to make sure that my long, beautiful curls are still there. I guess that trauma will never be erased from my memory—even all these years later.

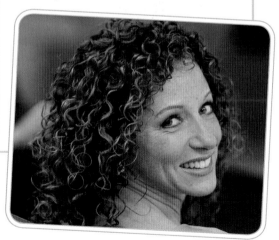

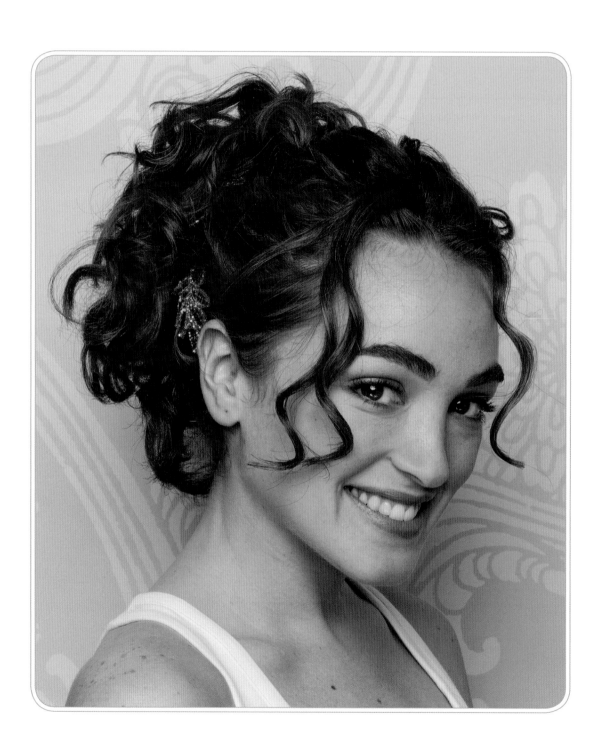

CHAPTER 3

identifying your curl type

Curls are like snowflakes or fingerprints. No two are alike, making it difficult to generalize about curly hair. Some of us are born with tightly coiled corkscrew curls so relentless that not even Superman could stretch them out, or so brittle that they break with the least resistance. Some of us have soft Botticelli curls that frame our face with ringlets, making us look like angels in Renaissance paintings. And millions of us have varying degrees of curls and waves and more than one type on one head. Some of us don't even know what our curl potential is. Your hair really will evolve once you know how to care for and style it. Waves turn into spirals, ringlets into corkscrews, and undefined fractal Afros into well-hydrated, shiny coils.

Curls are like a box of chocolates. You never know which type you're going to get.

There are many, many types of curl in this world (see page 30.) But to guide you in caring for your curls, I've categorized them into seven curl types: Corkscrew, Botticelli, and Corkicelli, Cherub, Wavy, S'wavy, and Fractal or Zigzag. To help you identify which curl type best matches your hair, I've used recognizable celebrities who represent each curl type along with that type's features and behaviors. Decide which celebrity and characteristics best match your hair, then go to the particular routine for your curl type in chapters 4 through 6 to learn how to nurture and encourage your curls.

CURLY CUE: THE SPRING FACTOR

The tightness of your curls (or spring factor) is a good way to determine which type of curly girl you are. (It's also something your hairdresser should know or be told because it tells him or her how much to cut.) The spring factor is the difference between the length of a curl when it falls naturally and when it's pulled out to its full length. Here's how to check yours: Pull a strand of dry curls down against your shoulder or neck to its full length. Leave your finger at the point where the strand touches. Now let go. With a ruler, measure the distance between your finger and where your curl naturally ends. The measurement is your personal spring factor:

9- to 16-inch spring: **Fractal** or **Zigzag**

9- to 12-inch spring: **Corkscrew**

5- to 10-inch spring: **Corkicelli** and **Cherub**

5- to 8-inch spring: **Botticelli**

2- to 4-inch spring: **Wavy**

1- to 2-inch spring: **S'wavy**

If you have short hair, your spring factor will be about half as long as the figures above.

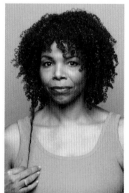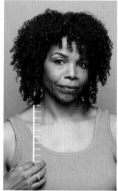

These fractal curls have about a 9-inch spring factor or more. Measure your spring factor to help determine which hair-care routine to follow.

DIFFERENT TYPES OF CURLS

Corkscrew Curls

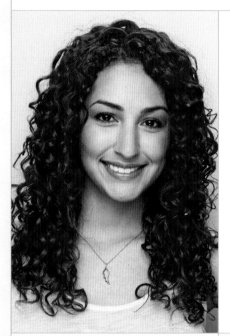

Sophia, Curly Girl Model

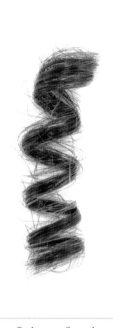

Corkscrew Sample

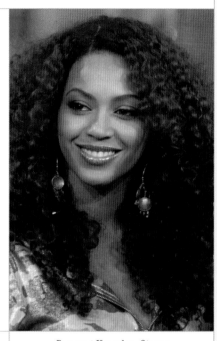

Beyoncé Knowles, Singer

You know you have corkscrew curls if you have:

- ☐ Curls that contract as tightly as a French poodle's if cut too short.
- ☐ Lots of small spirals.
- ☐ A high frizz factor.
- ☐ Hair that appears thickly textured when you look at it all together, but is actually baby-fine and delicate when you look at a single strand. (This is why your hair breaks so easily.)
- ☐ Hair that soaks up as much conditioner as you feed it.
- ☐ Tangles and snarls under the top layer of hair at the nape of the neck. (This is caused by the natural movement of the head throughout the day.)
- ☐ A spring factor of 9 to 12 inches.

DIFFERENT TYPES OF CURLS

Botticelli Curls

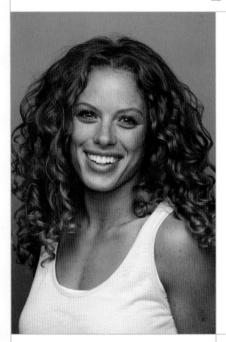

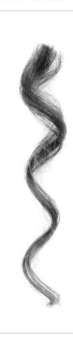

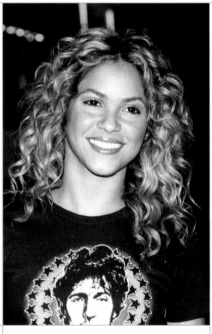

Jo, Curly Girl Model

Botticelli Sample

Shakira, Singer

You know you have botticelli curls if you have:

☐ Curls that vary in size and shape. Underneath you may have hermit curls that can shrink to half the length of those on the outside. (This is another reason *not* to cut your hair wet, something we'll discuss in chapter 9.)

☐ Curls that tend to be looser, in the shape of soft S's, combined with those that are tight.

☐ Curls that have a ropier appearance.

☐ Hair that seems to wilt if it gets too long. (This is because the weight of the top layer weighs the hair down.)

☐ Curls that are looser during some seasons and tighter during others.

☐ A spring factor of 5 to 8 inches.

DIFFERENT TYPES OF CURLS

Corkicelli Curls

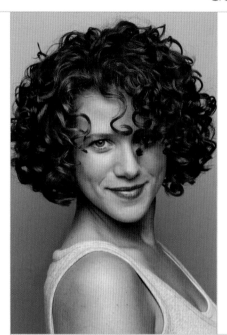

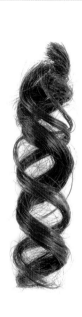

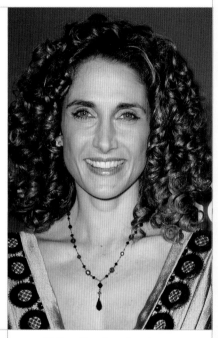

| Cyrille, Curly Girl Model | Corkicelli Sample | Melina Kanakaredes, Actress |

You know you have corkicelli curls if you have:

☐ Varying curl patterns throughout your hair's overall landscape: for example, significantly tighter curls around the face and at the nape of the neck, while the rest of the hair is much looser, or vice versa. (Curls should *never* be cut when wet, because you would not recognize these distinct curl patterns on a wet, combed surface.)

☐ Drier hair with a higher frizz factor if not hydrated properly.

☐ Curly hair throughout all seasons.

☐ Hair that appears longer or shorter depending on the weather and humidity.

☐ A spring factor of 5 to 10 inches.

Cherub Curls

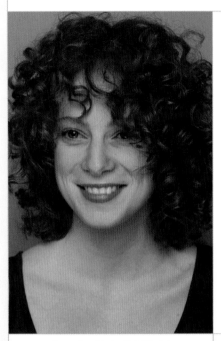

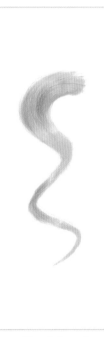

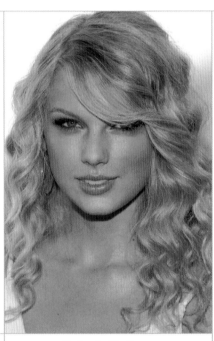

| *Lionelle, Curly Girl Model* | *Cherub Sample* | *Taylor Swift, Singer* |

You know you have cherub curls if you have:

☐ Had curly hair from birth.

☐ Baby-fine curl spirals that resemble the hair of a young child whether you're eight years old or eighty.

☐ Curls that seem as delicate as gold leaf because they easily disperse with outside interferences such as wind, moving around while you sleep, or too much touching.

☐ Curls that are weightless to the touch and have a translucency to them like a halo.

☐ A variety of curl lengths on your head.

☐ Curls that take a long time to grow and never seem to grow past a certain point. (Don't worry, they *will* grow with the right care.)

☐ Curls that have a shorter life span because they're so fragile that they break easily.

☐ A spring factor of 5 to 10 inches.

Wavy Hair

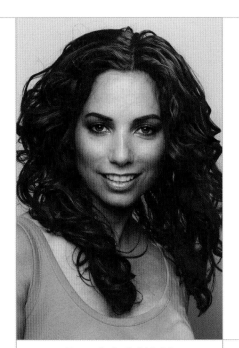

Erica, Curly Girl Model

Wavy Sample

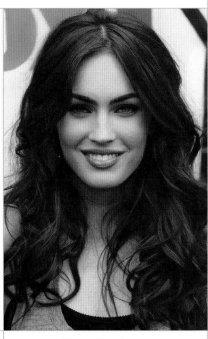

Megan Fox, Actress

You know you have wavy curls if you have:

- ☐ Hair that you've always believed was straight.
- ☐ Had straight hair when you were very young and possibly wavy hair after puberty.
- ☐ Hair that occasionally develops a natural wave after coming out of the shower and at the beach.

- ☐ A slight halo of frizz and frizz on the ends of the hair on humid days.
- ☐ Hair that has a tendency to look unmaintained and flat on the crown.
- ☐ Hair that can appear straight in the winter.
- ☐ Hair that is dry on the ends.
- ☐ A spring factor of 2 to 4 inches.

DIFFERENT TYPES OF CURLS

S'wavy Hair

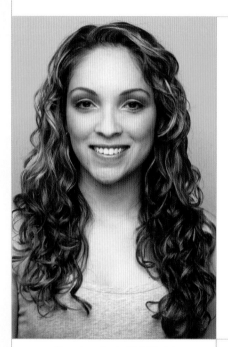

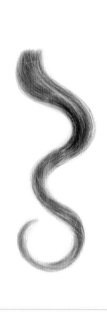

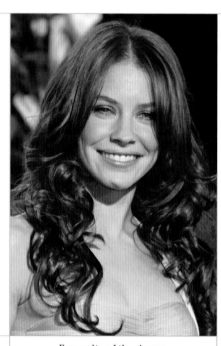

| *Carmine, Curly Girl Model* | *S'wavy Sample* | *Evangeline Lily, Actress* |

You know you have s'wavy curls if you have:

- ☐ Hair that may appear straight in the winter with no effort. In fact, you have to work to get waves in your hair. (Read on, because you can do it!)
- ☐ Low to no frizz factor.
- ☐ A natural shine.

- ☐ A slight bend at the ends of your hair, depending on the length.
- ☐ Hair that looks better when it's layered.
- ☐ A spring factor of 1 to 2 inches.

DIFFERENT TYPES OF CURLS

Fractal or Zigzag Curls

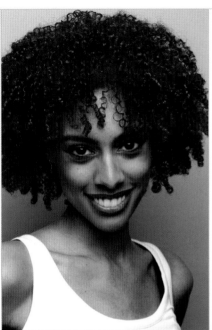

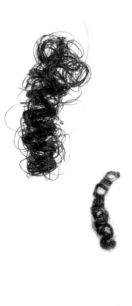

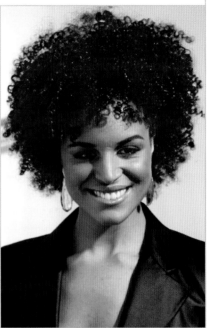

| *Olivia, Curly Girl Model* | *Fractal and Zigzag Samples* | *Laura Izibor, Singer* |

You know you have fractal or zigzag curls if you have:

☐ Curls that might be described as twizzles, micro-spirals, or fractal corkscrews.

☐ An almost steplike pattern to your hair. It may not look zigzag when you look at your hair as a whole, but it will when you take a closer look at individual curls.

☐ Hair that is relentlessly dry.

☐ Hair that's hypersensitive to rough handling.

☐ Curls that don't change with the season.

☐ A receding hairline from having your hair pulled back too tight, relaxed, or the weight of a weave. (All curly girls are prone to this, but fractal and zigzag curls are more so than others.)

☐ A spring factor of 9 to 16 inches.

curl confession

Faith Jones *feminist and writer*

L ike many African American little girls, I had my hair chemically relaxed when I was only four. When I got older, it was a constant battle between me and superstrength relaxers, straightening irons, blow-dryers, and plastic rollers. My life literally revolved around my hair. I scheduled my gym workouts around washing and roller-setting my hair, avoided swimming, and spent hours sweating under a hot hooded dryer, even in the summer. I would walk out of hair salons in tears from the painful chemical scalp burns.

The summer after my college graduation, during a Jamaican vacation, my hair was a frizzy, dry disaster from the sun and swimming. I considered going into town to have my hair braided, but I didn't want to spend seven hours doing it. Instead, I decided to enjoy my vacation, gross hair and all. I vowed to figure out a way to have this same carefree attitude about my hair when I got home. After searching for solutions, I realized the smartest thing to do was to grow out my relaxer. There were so many ways to transition from straight to curly hair, through straw-sets, braids, Bantu-knotting, and such. But after two months of transitioning, the effort these hairstyles took completely defeated the purpose of wanting carefree styling of my natural curls.

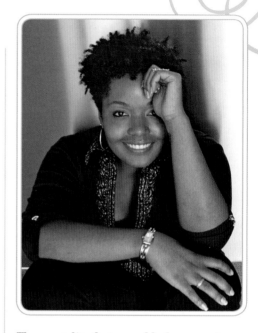

The mentality that many black women have about their hair is insane to me. Was I to spend the rest of my life battling with my hair to get it to do something it was never meant to do?

So I went to my hairstylist and had my hair cut off completely. I left happily bald-headed, the sun shining on my scalp, feeling truly liberated. Two years later, my hair is healthy, shiny, and wonderfully curly. After all those years of trying to obtain straight hair, I realized that all my hair needed was moisture and patience! I vowed once my virgin hair grew in that I'd never pollute it with harsh chemicals again.

YOU ARE WHAT YOU EAT—AND SO ARE YOUR CURLS

All hair benefits immensely from good nutrition. The health and radiance of your curls can be directly linked to your diet, says Esther Blum, RD, a New York–based registered dietician, holistic nutritionist, and author of *Eat, Drink, and Be Gorgeous: A Nutritionist's Guide to Living Well While Living It Up*. "In general, the diet for healthy hair is the diet for longevity," she says. Specifically, she recommends that you eat your protein. Since hair is 97 percent protein, you need this nutrient to help it grow and stay healthy. Just 2 to 3 ounces of protein three times per day is enough for the average person and 6 ounces three times per day if you're very physically active. Your healthiest bet is to eat free-range or organic protein because it doesn't contain hormones or antibiotics and, if possible, to eat meat from animals that are grass-fed.

Including healthy fats in your diet is important for shiny, thick locks. One of the first things you notice when a person has anorexia is dull, lifeless, thinning hair. Healthy fats keep your scalp hydrated, leaving your hair looking lush

DON'T SUFFOCATE YOUR HAIR WITH YOUR HANDBAG

I see so many long-haired women trap their curls beneath the straps of their shoulder bags. When they realize this, they unconsciously yank the trapped hair out from beneath the strap, ripping and fracturing their curls. Do this a few times every day for weeks and months and it will make one side of the hair appear weak and stringy. Remember to move your hair off your shoulders before slinging on your bag. And if hair does get stuck under the strap, first lift the bag off your shoulder and then move your hair.

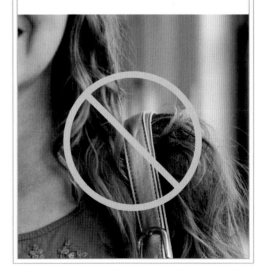

and shiny. Healthy fats include omega-3 essential fatty acids, which can be found in foods like avocado, ground flax seeds, flax seed oil, coconut oil, salmon, sardines, egg yolks, spinach, and walnuts, and include monounsaturated fats found in olives, olive oil, and nuts such as almonds and cashews. Trace minerals like zinc, magnesium, and selenium may help thinning hair or hair loss. You'll find them in raw nuts like almonds, walnuts, and cashews, seeds like pumpkin seeds, whole grains like brown rice, beans, and oats. To keep hair from thinning, be sure to get enough iron, which is plentiful in beef, turkey, eggs, and beans, and hyaluronic acid, which is found in chicken stock made from chicken bones.

CURL-OGRAPHY

Each curly head is a complex tonsorial topology containing many different curl formations. Here are the various curls that can happily coexist on one head:

▥ Canopy curls: The top layer of curls on your head, which suffer the most abuse from the environment and too much touching.

▥ Crouching curls: The protected layers of tightly coiled curls found close to the scalp and underneath the canopy. (I like to call them "crouching curls, hidden gorgeousness.")

▥ Halo: A loving word for the frizz around the crown of the head. You can tell whether you have a high or low frizz factor by how much halo you have.

▥ Hermit curls: Tight, coiled-back curls hiding near the nape of the neck that aren't obvious unless you pull them out and hold them down. Once you let go, they spring right back into hiding.

▥ East-west curls: Hair that balloons out on either side of the head but lies flat on top, making you look like the Sphinx or Gilda Radner's Roseanne Roseannadanna on *Saturday Night Live* (below).

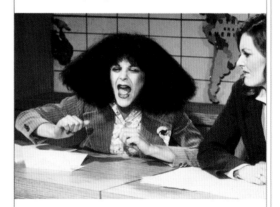

▥ North-south curls: Elongated by gravity, these curls hang longer.

curl confession

Shelley Ozkan *retail merchandiser*

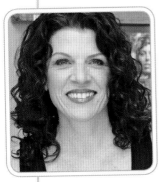

My first—and worst—hair trauma occurred when I was nine. I had very long, curly hair that fell halfway down my back, and I loved wearing it loose and carefree. My parents, who thought my hair looked unruly, announced that if I didn't start taking care of it, I'd have to get it cut off. One day, in the dead of winter, my mother made good on her threat and dragged me to a beauty parlor to get my hair cut in a short shag. I was so humiliated by the result that I decided to wear a knit cap to school until my hair grew back.

Don't even ask me what I went through in high school. It was the late seventies, when everyone but me had straight Farrah Fawcett hair. (I wonder if she had any idea how many curly girls suffered because of her hairstyle.) I'd wash my hair every night, blow-dry it straight, and pull it back in a ponytail. Then I'd wake up at 6 A.M. and wrap it around hot rollers to complete the straightening treatment. The day of my senior prom, I was even more obsessed than usual with the weather report. We lived in Pittsburgh, Pennsylvania, where it is very humid, and the May mist is a nightmare. I was wearing a to-die-for, off-the-shoulder gown, and I wanted my hair to be equally sleek. When I woke up that morning, the weather was hot and humid, and as the hours passed, the air remained laden with moisture. I gave up and let my hair do its thing.

When I emerged from my bedroom, my mother looked stunned. "Your hair looks beautiful," she said. "That's how you should always wear it." I was horrified by my hair. I'd imagined myself as Farrah Fawcett but I'd morphed into Shirley Temple.

When we arrived at the prom, I locked eyes across the ballroom with Mark, the boy I'd had a crush on since fourth grade. Like a scene from a movie, we walked toward each other, meeting halfway. "You look so beautiful," he said. "I can't believe what your hair looks like." We kissed passionately, right there in front of our dates. It was a magical moment. (Then he threw up all over his shoes. He was totally wasted. But he loved my hair.)

Today, I have two curly haired children and I'm so happy to say that they love their hair (my boys are pictured on page 130). I've been following the Curly Girl Method with them since they were born. Their hair has never been tortured with a blow-dryer and I've never used shampoo or a comb or brush. In fact, since my husband is curly, too, we don't have a comb or brush in our entire house!

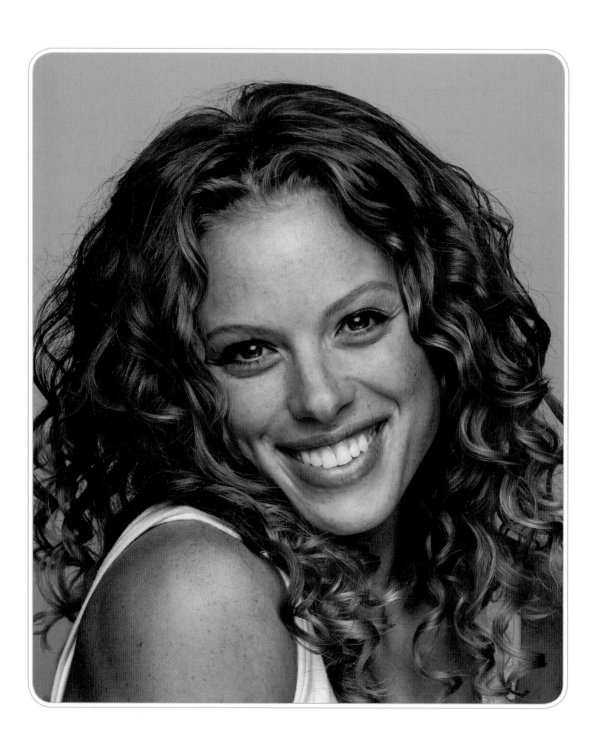

CHAPTER 4

the curly girl method

CREATING A DAILY ROOT-INE

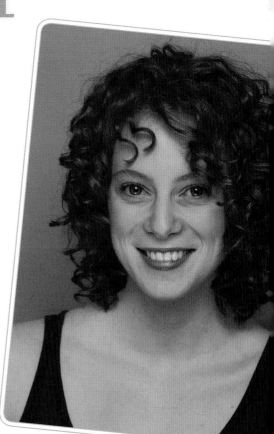

The place most curly girls go wrong is in the cleansing and styling of their hair. Of course, *all* the information in this book is important for gorgeous, healthy hair, but if you read just one chapter intently, it should be this one. That's because the most important part of loving and accepting your curls starts in the shower. Adopting this regimen of daily hair care means you'll have to unlearn a lot of assumptions you have about what constitutes "good" hair grooming, like using shampoo or the notion that you step in the shower and immediately start

SHAMPOO
=
SHAM (trick)
+
POO (the nasty stuff)
Go No-poo!

fussing with your locks. But I guarantee this curly girl approach will change your life with your hair.

The first unorthodox step is to throw out every bottle of shampoo in the bathroom and get rid of your blow-dryer (unless you use it with a diffuser, which we'll talk about on page 55), flat irons, brushes, and hot combs! I'm going to show you how to keep your hair and scalp clean with sulfate-free cleansers or, if you can't find a sulfate-free cleanser, a botanical conditioner (yes, you can cleanse with a conditioner).

Once you break your shampoo dependency, you'll still be rinsing and cleaning your hair regularly, but in a way that will keep it hydrated and healthy. The harsh detergents found in most shampoos strip hair of its lubrication and cause the hair's cuticle to stand straight up like guards at the gate, so things like dirt and product buildup can't get out. Curly hair is a dry, porous surface, so it holds onto the detergent-filled shampoo like a sponge, which is why it's so hard to fully rinse it all out. This is a disaster for organic hair fiber—especially curly hair!

Instead, sulfate-free cleansers and botanical conditioners soften and protect the hair. They keep the hair's cuticle

THere's no such THING as a LITTLE BLOW-DrYING . . .

A lot of curly girls think that blow-drying and flat-ironing their hair straight once in a while is okay. But it's not. Straightening your curls occasionally is like smoking a cigarette every once in a while—you'd be surprised how much damage can be done from just that once! It takes a while for curls to take shape and just be, and even one blow-fry or flat-ironing can set you back. Over time and with good care, the memory of the curl locks in, the frizz disappears, and your curls elongate. You're on auto-curl pilot and you don't want to derail it!

closed during the cleansing process, which prevents tangling and matting, and allow whatever is in your hair to exit easily when rinsing. Some curly girls may question whether they can truly clean their hair and scalp without sudsy shampoo. But I promise that the method I suggest—firmly massaging the entire surface of your scalp using circular motions—will get your scalp and hair clean.

The friction of your fingertips combined with cleanser or conditioner will loosen and break up dirt and product buildup, leaving the scalp cleansed and deodorized and your curls undisturbed, but clean. After all, friction is a time-tested method of cleaning (think of a washing machine churning). The massaging motion also stimulates blood flow to the scalp, which brings nutrients to the hair follicles, helping hair to grow and stay healthy.

In this chapter, you'll find out the cleansing and styling routines for these types of curly hair—corkscrew, botticelli, corkicelli, and cherub curls. Since wavy and s'wavy curls and fractal and zigzag curls have some different steps, each has a separate chapter. (For wavy and s'wavy, see chapter 5, Catching a Wave, page 51. For fractal and zigzag, see chapter 6, Multi-curl-tural Hair, page 61). However, the following general advice applies to all

curls and waves no matter how big, small, tightly wound, or loose.

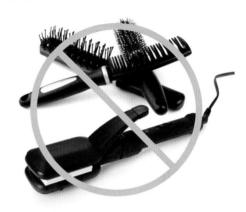

THE BASICS FOR

ALL TYPES OF CURLS

Whatever your type of curls, follow the general directions for cleansing, conditioning, scrunching, and styling your hair on the following spread. Also toss out your hairbrushes and combs, even those that claim to be made for curls. The act of brushing or combing the hair actually interferes with your curls' formation and causes breakage and dispersed curls—otherwise known as frizz! Instead, use your fingers to comb through the hair only when it's wet and drenched with conditioner in the shower. This way you respect each fragile curl's natural placement, and the hair is more fluid.

DIRT AGENTS

When I mention "cleanser" I always mean a sulfate-free cleanser, by "conditioner" I mean a botanical conditioner, and by "gel" I mean one that's free of harsh ingredients such as alcohol and silicone. I sometimes talk about cleanser and conditioner interchangeably because for some curly girls, using a conditioner is just as good as using a cleanser for cleaning. (See chapter 8, page 79, for pointers on how to read a hair-care ingredient label and how to determine which products are good or bad for your curls.)

THE BASICS FOR ALL TYPES OF CURLS

Cleansing

There are two parts to the cleansing routine for all curls: cleansing your scalp and hair and then conditioning your hair. How often you cleanse and condition depends on your hair and where you are in the process. If you're weaning yourself off shampoo, you may want to stay on your usual cleansing schedule, just replacing your regular shampoo with a sulfate-free product or a botanical conditioner. You might not like a bubble-free diet, but your hair will love it. Once your hair becomes more hydrated and healthy, you will probably cleanse less often and just wet your hair and go right to the conditioning step for your curl type. It's also important to allow the hair to rest at times and not get locked into a scheduled routine of overcleansing. I know wavy types who only wash their hair every three to four days.

If you are new to this curly girl approach to hair care, the amounts of product you use will change as your hair becomes healthier. For example, early on you may need to use lots of conditioner because your hair is dry and thirsty, then, as your hair gets hydrated, you'll use less. Because your curls' moods are so affected by weather and climate, you may have to adjust the amount of product you use when you travel or as the seasons change.

Generally, the tighter or drier the curl, the more botanical conditioner you need. Hair that's been damaged by blow-frying, coloring, or chemical straightening absorbs conditioner quickly and needs more. Experiment with different amounts to figure out what's best for your hair, but err on the side of more conditioner rather than less.

Conditioning

For most curl types, I suggest leaving some or all of your conditioner in your hair. I know this sounds unorthodox, especially since we're so conditioned—ahem!—to rinsing thoroughly for fear that product will weigh our hair down. But curly hair needs that extra moisture to stay hydrated and frizz-free, and the word greasy is almost never relevant to a curly girl. Others worry that leaving conditioner in will make your hair crunchy or sticky, but that won't happen with the right product (see chapter 8, page 79, for choosing a conditioner). In fact, a favorite trick of girls with a high frizz factor and dense, thick curls is to not rinse out any conditioner at all. Why? Because when you squeeze out excess water with a paper towel or microfiber towel (see photo, right), it's like rinsing—the hair naturally absorbs the conditioner it needs to stay hydrated and releases what it doesn't.

In the conditioning sections for each type of curl, I suggest gliding conditioner downward through your hair with your fingers. If you have longer hair, follow this step by scrunching the same section of hair upward toward the scalp. This opposite motion will encourage and reintroduce your intrinsic curl pattern to your hair.

I often use the words "squeeze-quench" to describe the process of squeezing hair with conditioner in an upward motion toward the scalp. It usually releases a milky residue of excess water and conditioner. A squishy sound and hair that feels as viscous as wet seaweed means that "hydration penetration" has been accomplished.

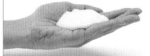

A generous palmful of conditioner gives curls frizz-fighting hydration.

THE BASICS FOR ALL TYPES OF CURLS

Scrunching

Never dry curls with a conventional towel, because it will absorb too much moisture and its harsh fabric will ruffle the sensitive hair cuticle, causing frizz. Instead, I suggest using a paper towel, an old cotton T-shirt, or a microfiber towel. Though I mention these three options throughout the book, you can use anything smooth and absorbent, like a pillowcase or baby's burp cloth. Gently rotate the fabric as you blot the hair. Just like blotting a sweater in a towel after washing, precious hair fibers need the same gentle care. "Scrunch-squeeze" is how I describe the upward scrunching motion toward the scalp that you make with a microfiber towel to absorb extra moisture.

Use a paper towel, an old cotton T-shirt, or a microfiber towel to absorb moisture from curly locks.

Styling

Gel is an important part of every curly girl's routine because it gives definitive hold but is light to the touch. As your hair begins to dry and the gel hardens, don't be alarmed by the crystallized curl cast, or "gel cast." This helps hold the natural curl formation until the hair dries, protecting it from outside elements like wind and humidity. Once hair is completely dry, you can dissolve and release the gel cast by tilting your head forward and gently scrunching hair upward toward the scalp. The result will be soft, defined, touchable curls. It's important to use a gel that's alcohol- and silicone-free, as it lives in your hair for 2 to 3 days.

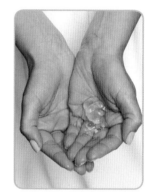

A half palmful of gel helps hold your curls' natural shape.

Note: For each type of curl in the book, I give an approximate time for how long it will take to cleanse and style. This period will get shorter as hair gets healthier and more hydrated.

Simply being curly is not enough. Beautiful, healthy hair is the result of first accepting your curls for their natural tendencies, then working with them, and being really consistent in your daily care routine. Remember, you are the custodian of that little garden atop your head! It will reflect the care that you give it.

DAILY ROUTINE FOR

BOTTICELLI, CORKSCREW, AND CORKICELLI CURLS

■ **Total cleansing/conditioning and styling time:** 10 to 15 minutes, depending on the length of the hair.

Cleansing and Conditioning

1 Step under the shower as if you're standing under a waterfall and let the water cascade through your curls. Resist the impulse to start scrubbing your head and disturbing your hair's basic shape. If the water pressure is strong, cup your hair in your hands. Wet hair thoroughly.

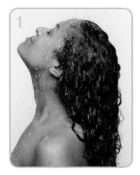

2 Cup one hand, take a sulfate-free cleanser or botanical conditioner, and apply it in a straight line along your fingertips the way you'd apply toothpaste to a toothbrush. Evenly distribute to the fingertips of the other hand and then apply directly to the scalp; be careful not to disturb your curls.

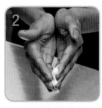

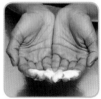

Distribute cleanser evenly on fingertips.

3 Starting at the temples, massage the scalp with circular motions, move down the sides and then to the top of your head and crown. Finally, move down the back of your head, finishing up at the nape. Now let the water spray through your hair, rinsing out whatever your

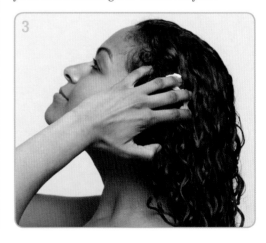

HaLO GOOD-BYe

In the past, you probably shampooed the top of your hair first. It is usually the first place to get rinsed, too, so conditioner was washed out before it did its job. No wonder we curly girls have been f.b.i. (frizz-bewildered individuals) for years. We need to reverse this sequence: Have the top of your head be the last place you apply cleanser and the last place you rinse out conditioner. And say good-bye to your frizz halo forever.

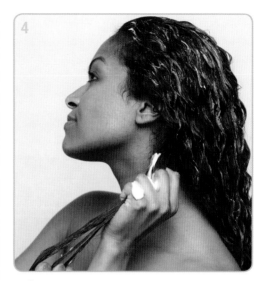

fingers have loosened. When you rinse the top of your hair, the ends of the hair will get clean as the cleanser or conditioner moves downward. This method will create fewer tangles and will prevent overwashing the typically drier, more mature ends of your hair.

4 Take a generous palmful of your conditioner (see page 36), evenly distribute it between your hands, and graze it downward on the outer layer (aka the canopy) of your hair as if you were icing a cake. If needed, apply more conditioner through the hair at each side of your head, using your fingers as a comb. The point is to distribute the conditioner evenly through your hair's landscape so no curl is left behind. Now your hair should feel smooth and silky— like wet seaweed.

5 Apply a dollop of conditioner (about the size of a quarter) under the hair at the nape of your neck, the spot most prone to tangles and knots. The hair there breaks easily, so be patient and gentle when trying to release any tangles or knots with your fingers. (Ripping equals frays and frays equal more knots.) Then, using your

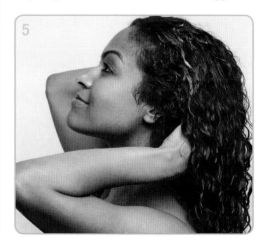

fingers, comb through your hair from underneath, removing any loose hairs. Remember, it's normal to lose about a hundred strands a day!

6 Before rinsing your hair, stand away from the shower flow. Cup your hands under the water and splash water over your hair a couple of times. I call this a trickle or baptism rinse; it ensures that the canopy of the hair, which is constantly exposed to the environment and thus very dry, can have the right amount of conditioner to stop it from frizzing. Over time, you'll know instinctively whether to rinse out any more conditioner at this point. If you do rinse, just let the shower spray fall over your head for a few seconds to evenly distribute the conditioner without removing it.

Styling

1 Step out of the shower and tilt your head forward. Loosely cupping a microfiber towel, paper towel, or an old cotton T-shirt, gently squeeze upward toward the scalp to remove excess water and encourage curl formation (see page 37). (It should sound very squishy.) Repeat this motion all around your head. If you like your curls to be fuller, do this until the hair no longer drips; if you want more gravity to your curls, leave in more water.

2 With the head still tilted forward, let your curls fall freely. Place a palmful of gel in one hand and evenly distribute it to the other hand. Apply the gel evenly throughout the landscape of the hair, making sure you cover all your curls. Starting at the ends, scrunch sections of hair up toward the scalp (visualize that you're pushing a spring together with both hands, and then releasing it). This method will cultivate or enhance the curl formation.

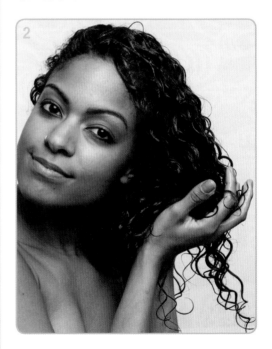

3 Slowly raise your head to an upright position, look up at the ceiling, and gently shake your hair so your curls fall

into their natural position. If it's a humid day or you have a high halo frizz factor, take an additional quarter-sized amount of gel and rub it in both hands. Then very gently graze the gel over the top layer of hair so the cuticle will be smooth.

GET a GRIP: THE CLIPPING TECHNIQUE

The roots of curly hair can sometimes dry flat because of the weight of the wet hair pulling downward. This is especially the case with longer hair. Clipping hair at the roots relieves the wet hair of its own weight as it dries, so you add lift and get a more even curl pattern from roots to ends. This also helps hair dry faster. Here's how to use clips:

1. Place clips along the part where the roots meet the scalp. If you place the clip farther down the hair, you'll add more weight and make the roots flatter. Don't be afraid of doing it wrong; it's really very simple if you don't overthink it. Using a clawlike motion, lift a small amount of hair from the top of your head. (The hair should be gently pulled perpendicular to the scalp, not forward or backward.) Open the clip, slide it in at the base of the hair and leave it. Make sure the hair is as tight as when you pinched it and that the clip is close to the scalp. You will need about six clips to lift the top of your hair—in front, at the crown, and between those two points. Now leave your hair alone and let it dry.

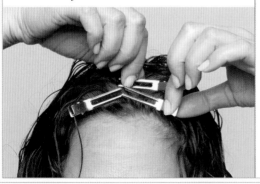

2. For a little more advanced clipping, you may want to target areas where your hair tends to get flat when it dries, like the sides of the head at the area where the head curves near the crown (where a cowlick would be). As hair gets longer, this flat spot is more apparent, and if you color your hair, it's where your roots show first. Use a side mirror to help you find your target for clipping. After some practice, you'll be able to do this without looking.

3. Once your hair dries completely, use care and patience to remove the clips because hair swells during drying and can wrap around the clip the way ivy wraps around a tree trunk. To take clips out, anchor the piece of hair gently with one hand, then with the other hand, open the clip and slide it out.

4. Sometimes you may want to leave the clips in for extra styling lift all day. If the clips are the same color as your hair, no one can see them hidden in your curls once your hair dries. For a greater lift, add gel to the clips.

SPOT CLEANSING

Spot cleansing your hair can be done as often as you like. Just spray lavender mist (see chapter 8, page 83, for the spray recipe) on a soft but durable damp paper towel and wind it around your fingertip. Place your paper towel-clad finger on the scalp. With firm, circular motions, rub out all dirt particles as you would a stain on a shirt. For wigs, extensions, and weaves you can use the same paper towel-covered finger technique, by gliding over the surface and moving downward while lightly pressing. This cleaning method is also great to use when you are traveling or camping.

4 To give the curls on the top of your head a little volume, you need to "lift and clip" the hair at the roots. This method releases the top layer of hair from its own weight, allowing it to dry faster and in an even curl pattern from roots to ends. (For the clipping technique, see page 41.) Don't interrupt the curls while they're drying or they'll frizz up.

5 If you don't have time to air-dry your hair, you can use a diffuser (see page 55), hooded dryer (they're surprisingly inexpensive and portable), or, if you're on the go, just put the heater on in your car. This creates the same kind of drying microclimate that you'd get from a hooded dryer.

6 When your hair is completely dry, remove the clips *very* gently, to prevent them from ripping hair. Lean over, place your hands on your scalp, and with the tips of your fingers, very lightly shake your hair at the roots to open up the curls. Stand upright, and very gently lift your fingers off the scalp, *not* raking them through your hair (which can cause frizz). **Note:** Skip this step if you like a more contained curl.

curl confession

Beth Pilar *co-owner of How Sweet It Is cake shop, New York City*

When I was seven, I was obsessed with Dorothy Hamill's haircut—that shiny bowl cut with bangs that she sported when she skated her way to an Olympic Gold Medal. I begged my mom to let me get a similar cut, and though she gently tried to discourage me (because she knew it wouldn't work with my very curly hair), I persisted. Finally, she gave in and took me to the salon. I showed the hairstylist the Dorothy Hamill photos that I'd cut out of magazines. The stylist and my mother exchanged glances, as if they were agreeing to let me get this haircut just to show me it wouldn't work. And they were right.

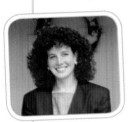

To replicate that famous bowl cut, I had to blow-dry my hair each morning. (Yes, a seven year old blow-drying her hair each morning before school!) It would look good initially, but after twenty minutes, it was all downhill. I'd return home from school with a short, frizzy mess. I was so mad at my hair, wondering why it wouldn't do what I wanted after so much hard work.

In fifth grade, my family moved from the city to a suburb. As if switching schools midyear wasn't traumatic enough, I was devastated to find that all the girls wore their hair in long, straight ponytails—something I coveted to no end. Then I met Kim, a classmate, who, along with her sister, had the best hair. Every day at 6:30 A.M., I'd bike to Kim's house, where she'd slather my hair in products, blow it straight, and slick it into one of those long ponytails. Still, there was always something gnawing at me—this anxious feeling that my hair could change with the weather or, worst of all, at swim class! I actually love swimming, but the thought of how my hair would look after class made it a horrible experience.

In junior high, a friend who had hair I thought was like mine, got an adorable short, wavy-curly haircut. I decided to give up my long, straight ponytail and do the same. My friend's haircut was cute; mine was horrible. It looked like a giant Brillo pad sitting on my head.

Finally, during a hippie phase in college, I let my hair go natural and loved it. Now I regret all the time and agony I wasted wrestling with my curls. But I also learned a bigger lesson: Don't try to make yourself fit an image that doesn't make sense for you. This is who I am, curly hair and all!

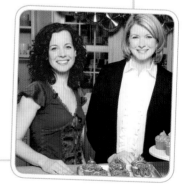

DAILY ROUTINE FOR

CHERUB
CURLS

■ Total cleansing/conditioning and styling
time: 6 to 10 minutes.

Cleansing and Conditioning

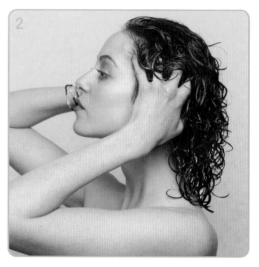

1 Stand under the shower and cup your hair so the water flowing through it doesn't disrupt or straighten the formation of this delicate curl type. Resist the impulse to start scrubbing your head and disturbing your hair's basic shape. Wet hair thoroughly.

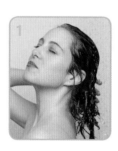

2 Cherub curls do not need as much cleanser as other curl types because they're so baby-fine and too much product can weigh them down. Cup one hand and apply a mounded tablespoon of sulfate-free cleanser or botanical conditioner along the pads of your fingers, and evenly distribute the cleanser to the fingertips of the other hand.

Starting at the temples, use firm circular massaging motions down the sides of your head, then move to the top of the head going gently toward the crown. Finally, move down the back of your head, finishing up at the nape.

3 Rinse your hair by cupping it in your hands and allowing the water to flow through your fingers like a sieve.

SCALP TREATMENT
(FOR ALL HAIR TYPES)

Once a week, give your scalp an exfoliating scrub treatment. Exfoliating will slough off any dead skin cells and product buildup, making your scalp healthier and relieving any itchiness. See chapter 8, page 84, for exfoliating scrub recipe and directions.

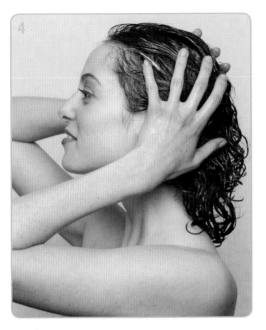

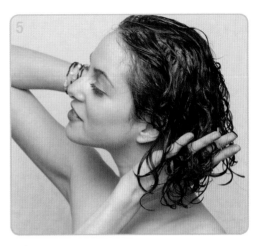

4 Take a generous amount of botanical conditioner and evenly distribute it between your hands. Apply it to the entire canopy of the hair making sure no curl is left behind.

5 Apply a dollop of conditioner about the size of a quarter underneath, to the hair at the nape of your neck. Even though Cherub curls are a very delicate hair type, they require lots of hydration to stay flexible and prevent breakage. Then gently comb your fingers through your curls from underneath, removing any loose hairs. Don't be concerned when you come away with strands in your hand; it's normal to lose many hairs a day!

6 Stand away from the shower's water stream, cup your hands under the water, and splash it over your hair a couple of times. This "trickle rinse" method ensures that you don't remove too much conditioner from the canopy of the hair, which needs extra hydration because of its constant exposure to the elements. If you're looking for more volume to your hair, rinse conditioner out of the hair more thoroughly by standing under the water stream while cupping your hair in your hands. (In this case, put in extra gel to secure and hold the curl formation during the drying process.)

SKIP THE CONDITIONER

If your cherub curls are well-hydrated, you may not need to condition them after cleansing.

Styling

1 Step out of the shower. With a paper towel, microfiber towel, or an old cotton T-shirt, scrunch-squeeze sections of hair upward, tilting your head from side to side.

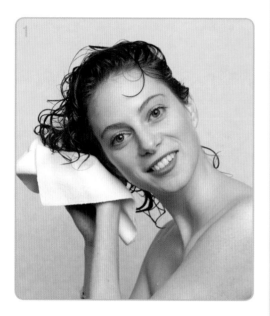

2 If you've used the trickle rinse and left conditioner in your hair, bring your head to an upright position and look up to the ceiling. Shake your hair back and forth to help your curls settle into place. Take a shallow palmful of gel, evenly distribute it in both hands, and very lightly graze down the canopy to ensure that every curl is covered.

3 If you rinsed out most of the conditioner, keep your head tilted forward after scrunch-squeezing your hair. Take a generous palmful of gel, evenly distribute it to both hands, and squeeze it into the hair from the bottom of the curl toward the scalp in an upward motion, making sure every curl is covered. Bring head upright, and shake it gently back and forth to help your curls settle into place. If your hair has a high frizz factor, take a tiny bit more gel and graze it gently down the canopy of the hair.

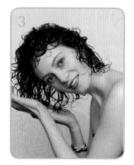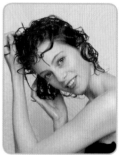

Squeeze gel from bottom of the curl toward the scalp as if you were pushing a spring together.

4 Cherub curls tend to get flat at the roots so you may want to use a few clips along the part of the hair to get some lift. Using a clawlike motion, lift a small amount of hair along the part (hair should be pulled perpendicular to the scalp, not forward or backward). Place a clip at the roots where you pinched the hair and at a right angle to the scalp. Any higher along

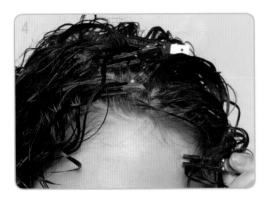

the hair and the clips will weigh it down, making the roots look even flatter. You'll need about four to six clips.

5 Cherub curls also tend to contract a lot, especially in the hair around your face, so you may want to place a clip at the

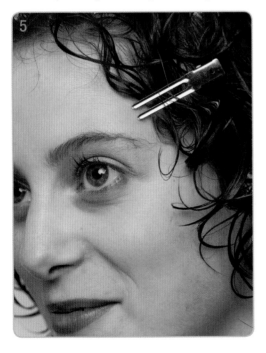

DO NOT DISTURB

When your curls are drying, they can be dispersed or frizzed by ruffling winds, fingers, combs and brushes, as well as by putting on and taking off clothes. So after styling your hair, keep your hands away from your curls as you let them dry. Also, if you're new to being a curly girl, don't run your fingers through your hair when it's dry and don't let others do it either. If you want to give curls a lift during the day, aerate them rather than raking your fingers through your curls. Here's how: With your head tilted forward, lightly place your hands on your scalp and gently shuffle your fingers at the roots. Keeping your hands in your scalp, slowly stand upright and shuffle your fingers a little more. Then very, very gently lift your fingers off the scalp without raking them through the hair. This last step is very important or else you'll disrupt your curls.

ends of your wet bangs or other short pieces to weigh them down while drying so they appear longer.

6 It's best to let your cherub curls air dry, because they are so fragile and heat can sometimes evaporate the gel. But if you don't have time, dry it with a diffuser (see page 55), a hooded dryer, or, if you're on the go, just put the heater on in your car.

7 When your hair is completely dry, remove the clips very gently. Tiny hairs may wrap around the clips during the drying process, and gentle handling prevents them from ripping or snapping.

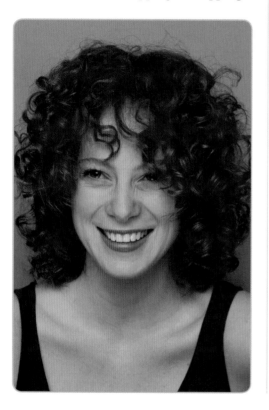

LOCK 'N' ROLL

If you don't feel like going through your usual hair care routine in the morning, a lavender spray (see page 83 for a homemade recipe) can refresh your curls quickly and reactivate the gel in the hair from the previous day. Tilt your head to one side, spray hair with the lavender spray, and scrunch hair gently upward toward the scalp. Tilt your head to the other side and repeat. Do so in the back as well. If you have any curls that have become dispersed overnight, spritz them with the lavender spray, twist them around your finger, slide the hair off your finger, and then clip the curl horizontally at the root. Let hair dry for 5 to 20 minutes, then carefully remove any clips. Shake your head, gently loosen hair at scalp with your fingers, and go.

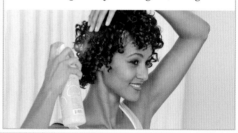

curl confession

Jo Newman *actress*

I had gotten used to my curls, imposed a self-taught regimen to keep the frizz at bay, and was finally beginning to feel comfortable in my skin—I mean hair—when I moved to New York City to launch my acting career. The first photographer I found to take my head shots panicked when I showed up at his studio. "No one will ever hire you with that hair," he said. "Name one famous actress with curly hair that wild." This was 2001, when Hollywood's women seemed to be competing for the straightest locks in the land; when the *Friends* girls appeared to be sleeping with their hot irons more than their boyfriends, and the new Japanese hair-straightening system was all the rage at my hair salon.

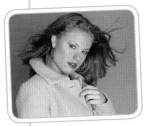

The straight-haired head shot that didn't land Jo as many acting gigs.

I was determined to be a success and wasn't going to let my hair get in the way of my career. But I cried when I got the photos back. They looked like someone else; someone boring, passive, and vulnerable. In one, he even had me in a wig. But I had them printed and sent off to every agency in the book. Apparently I was not the only one who didn't like my photos. No one called.

Two years later, I learned about the Curly Girl Method. I stopped shampooing and discovered clips. I had new headshot photos taken, this time with my hair natural. I sent them out, and I began getting work immediately. I was in many dressing rooms with other girls who would be fighting the humidity with brushes and serums and thousands of watts of electricity, but not once did anyone pull out a staightening iron or ask me to hide my curls. We would always end up talking about curls. Out of my element, but at home in my curls, I was on the way to finding myself.

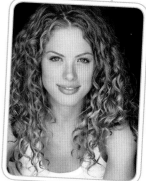

Head shot with natural curls. Much better!

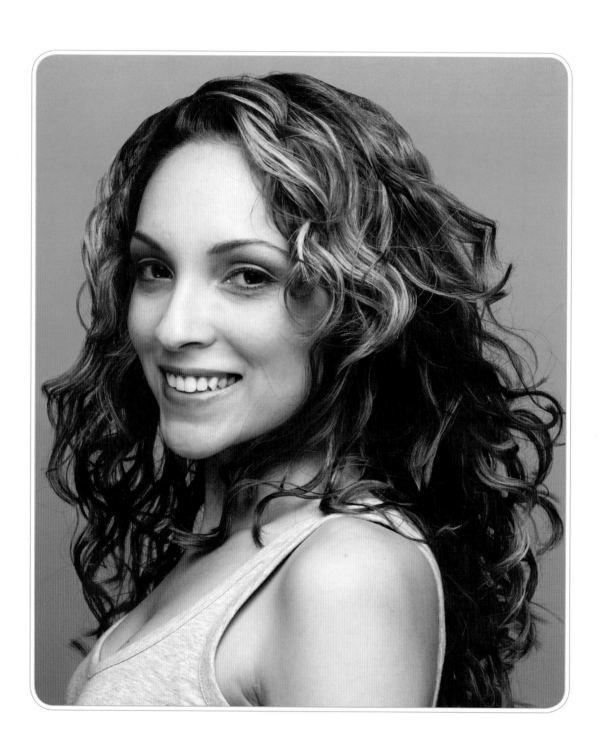

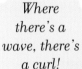

CHAPTER 5

catching a wave

Girls with wavy and s'wavy hair are often the most misunderstood and underrecognized types because their hair can easily be confused for straight. Wavy hair lies flat against the scalp, and every curl is in the shape of an S. Some are very loose, floppy S's while others are more defined. Some wavy hair may have a spring factor of 5 inches, while other waves fall in extremely lazy S's below the shoulders and barely spring at all. Very often, the hair has to grow past the shoulders before S shapes can appear and then begin to twist and turn. Wavy girls who think they are straight may be on too strict a diet of frequent haircuts, downward brushing, and blow-drying, so that the waves are attacked before they have a chance to reveal themselves. If hair is short, the wave or curl may not even be discernible.

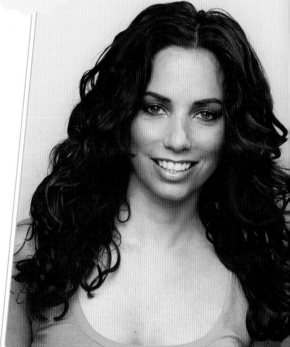

Though wavy hair isn't usually as dry as really curly locks can be, you should still toss every bottle of shampoo in your bathroom and cleanse with a sulfate-free cleanser or botanical conditioner. You should also stop using a blow-dryer or flat iron and never use a brush. When it comes to how often you should wash your hair, you'll need a little trial and error to figure it out. Often by the second or third day without cleansing, this sensitive hair type has more movement and body. Many of my wavy and s'wavy girls lightly cleanse only every three to four days and, between cleansings, they revive their hair with a spritz of lavender.

I urge you not to have so many self-imposed rules. If your hair still looks great after a few days without cleansing, *leave it alone!* Give it another day or two before washing and you might be surprised at the beautiful contours you see! A lot of caring for wavy and s'wavy hair is about what you're *not* going to do, rather than what you do.

Treat your hair gently and properly by following the cleansing and styling directions here and encourage your natural wave. After three weeks, you may be surprised to discover your full wavy potential with loose, glamorous curls that shine with good health.

DAILY ROUTINE FOR
WAVES AND S'WAVES

■ **Cleansing/conditioning and styling time:**
8 to 12 minutes, depending on length of hair.

Cleansing and Conditioning

1 Step under the shower's running water, cupping your hair with your hands so the water pressure does not leave your waves limp and lethargic. (If the water pressure is very high, try to lower it on the shower nozzle.) If you have baby-fine waves, put on a hairnet (available at Sally Beauty Supply) before you go under the water. The net allows water to flow through and lets you cleanse hair with your fingers while helping to contain your hair's wave structure.

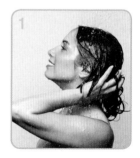

2 Cup one hand and apply a sulfate-free cleanser or botanical conditioner to the pads of your fingers. Evenly distribute the cleanser to the fingertips of

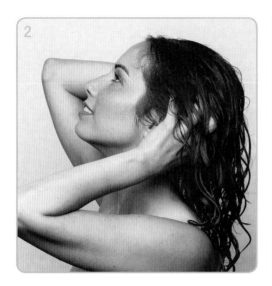

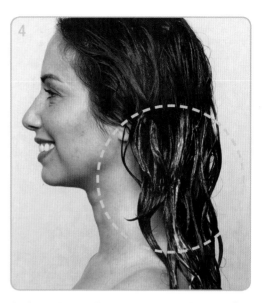

Apply conditioner beginning at the midsection of your hair.

the other hand. Starting at the temples, use firm, circular motions of your fingertips to rub your scalp gently down the sides. Then move to the top of your head, massaging toward the crown. Finally, move down the back of your head, finishing up at the nape. (To make waves and s'waves look thicker, see page 55.)

3 Let the shower spray run through your hair, rinsing out whatever dirt and product build-up your fingers have loosened. Cup your hair in your hands as you rinse and squeeze upward at the same time so you hear a squishy sound.

4 Take a shallow palmful of botanical conditioner and apply it from the midsection of your hair to the ends. Applying it to the roots can make hair too

limp. The only exception is if you tend to have a halo of flyaways at the roots. In that case, put a small amount of conditioner on your fingertips and graze it lightly over the canopy of the hair. Low frizz-factor wavy hair or baby-fine shorter hair may not always need conditioning after cleansing. It may make your hair too soft and reduce its body. Experiment with both methods. And if your hair feels well hydrated after cleansing, skip the conditioner and go to the styling section.

5 From the roots to the ends, comb conditioner through the hair with your fingers to smooth the cuticle and gather any loose hairs. Then take those

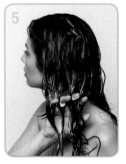

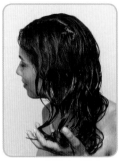

same sections and scrunch upward. This opposite motion after combing will nurture and encourage your hair's wave pattern.

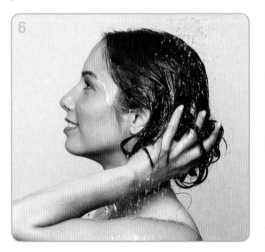

6 Cup your hair in your hands while standing under the water stream and rinse the hair thoroughly. Though other curl types leave some or all of their conditioner in the hair, wavy types should rinse it out completely so the weight of the conditioner doesn't leave wavy strands flat.

Styling

1 Lean over at the waist and tilt your head forward. Cup your hair loosely with a microfiber towel, paper towel, or an old cotton T-shirt and scrunch-squeeze as much water out of your hair as possible.

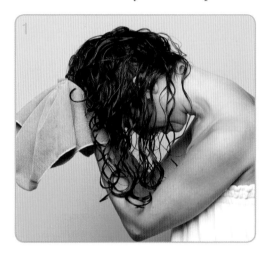

2 In the same tilted position, evenly distribute a shallow palmful of gel to both hands and coat your hair with the gel, using the scrunch-squeeze method.

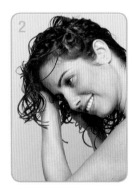

3 For a subtle lift at the crown, clip hair at the roots before diffusing it. (For clip tips, see chapter 4, page 41.) Clipping

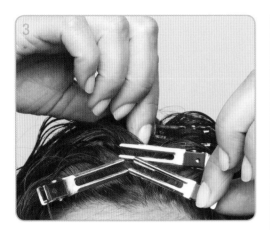

at the roots relieves the wet hair of its own weight as it dries. Add a little gel to the clip and leave it in until hair is completely dry.

4 Then you have three options for making waves. You may want to experiment to see which gives you the waves you crave, or use them at different times to achieve a variety of looks.

▧ Bring your head upright and gently shake waves into their natural position and let them air dry. This is best for more defined waves rather than loose ones.

▧ Keep your head tilted over and use a blow-dryer with a diffuser on a low to medium setting, or sit under a hooded dryer. Both are good techniques for wavy and s'wavy girls because it dries the hair faster and locks in the gel, helping the

waves form with definition and hold. It also prevents the water and gel from weighing down the waves.

▧ Place a yoga mat on the floor, and put a towel over it. Then lie down on the mat and spread your wet, gelled locks open on the floor around your head like a veil. Dry your hair with a diffuser set on low. Because the hair is resting on the floor, not being pulled down by gravity, its weightlessness guarantees body without frizz. A friend does this and her hair always looks full and amazingly defined.

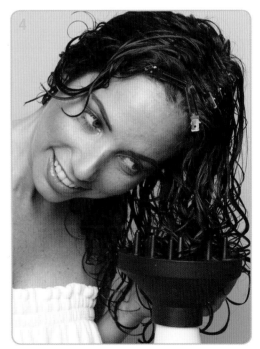

For wavy and s'wavy curls, try drying your hair with a diffuser set on low to medium.

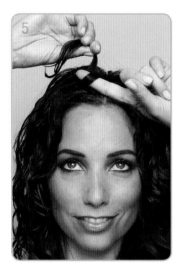
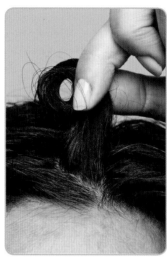
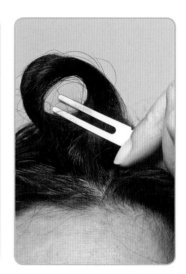

5 On dry or second-day hair, if you want a curlier look, try the pin curl method. Starting at the crown, wrap a section of hair around your finger, slide your finger out, hold the coil with your other hand, and insert a clip at a right angle. (The pin curls should stand out from your head, not lie flat.) Put all of your hair in giant pin curls. After the hair is dry, gently remove the clips by holding the hair with one hand and opening the clip with the other. Loosen your curls with your fingers.

6 Tilt your head forward and scrunch hair to loosen the gel cast (see page 58). Spritz hair with a spray gel for extra hold, if desired.

Re-FResH-meNt foR YouR cuRls

It's the end of a busy day and you're heading for a night out. But you're leaving in less than ten minutes and have no products or clips with you. Don't disp-hair! Wet your hands in the sink, tilt your head forward, and scrunch upward, which should reactivate the gel that's already in your hair. If you're looking for more volume, shuffle your curls at the scalp (see chapter 4, page 42). If you have any dispersed curls, wet a finger, wind the curl around it, and hold it for a minute. Repeat this on any curls, as needed. You will be amazed at how quickly your hair can revive!

WEATHER YOU'RE WAVY OR S'WAVY

If you're a wavy or s'wavy girl, you've probably noticed that the amount of wave or curl you have changes with the seasons and climate. In humid areas and in summer, your waves and s'waves are probably well defined, whereas in arid locales, such as desert areas, or in winter, wavy and s'wavy hair can appear almost straight if you do nothing to it. A few things can help in caring for your curls in wintertime or when you are in dry climates:

▨ In arid areas like the desert, a water filter attached to your showerhead is a must. Water tends to be harder in these regions and can leave a gummy residue on the hair.

▨ To add extra body to hair, mix gel with your sulfate-free cleanser. Cleanse as directed on page 52 and rinse well. Scrunch and squeeze with a microfiber towel. Then apply gel again for styling (This really works!) Also, using a hairnet in the shower can keep your wave formation intact.

▨ Add extra gel while styling to provide more hold throughout the day. Gel evaporates more quickly in the winter.

▨ For a sure hold, allow the product cast to stay firm and let it dissolve and open naturally during the day.

▨ Using a blow-dryer with a diffuser or hooded dryer on a medium heat setting can help hair dry more quickly and lock in the curl formation. In this case, use extra gel because the heat will evaporate it. You might want to use a spray gel after drying your hair.

▨ Get a top-grade humidifier for your home. This will encourage your curls, and also keep skin from drying out.

▨ Spritz hair with lavender spray mixed with gel (see page 80 for spray-gel recipe) to uplift waves on mornings when you don't cleanse your hair or to revive waves during the day.

▨ If you don't plan to cleanse your hair the next morning, preserve the formation of your waves by spritzing lightly with spray gel and balling your hair into a bun on the top of your head for the night. Unfurl the next morning.

THE GEL CAST— CLOSED AND OPEN

When your styling gel dries, it crystallizes to set the curl formation— this is why I keep reminding you not to touch your hair while it is drying. In the photograph below, the hair on the left still has a gel cast; the looser, fuller hair on the right has been scrunched to release the cast. The best way to open or loosen the gel cast is to tilt your head to the side or forward and gently scrunch the hair toward the scalp. Do this all around the head.

If you have a big event planned for the evening, you might want to leave in the gel cast all day at work to maintain the set, then release it right before the special occasion. Leaving in the gel cast also helps preserve the hair if it's raining.

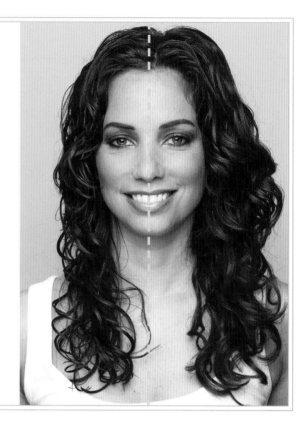

curl confession

Jessica Lamb-Shapiro *writer*

My first hair trauma happened when I was eight. My new stepmother thought my curly hair looked messy and was too hard to comb, so she took me to get my hair cut. I wanted to keep it long, but she wanted to have it all cut off, so we compromised: It would be short in front and long in the back. Little did I know I was asking for the infamous haircut known as a mullet! I burst into tears, and wore a scarf on my head until it grew out.

In college, I saved all my extra money to treat myself to a haircut at a fancy Fifth Avenue salon in New York City. I was convinced that I was going to get a fabulous haircut—that was until I sat down in the hairstylist's chair and she said, dismayed, "I don't know how to cut your hair. They only taught us how to cut straight hair." Then she had a brainstorm: "I'll blow-dry your hair, and then cut it!" Even straight, the haircut wasn't great; as soon as I washed it, it was a disaster.

My own attempts to blow-dry my hair were a joke. The best I could come up with was to put my wet hair in a ponytail, so that the top would dry straight and the bottom would dry curly. This made me look a bit as though I'd stuck my finger into an electrical socket, but it was better than nothing.

Then a friend told me about a curly hair salon. The very idea was strange to me, as if it wasn't a salon if everyone didn't come out looking like a Pantene commercial. But I loved my friend's hair, so I thought I would give it a shot. When I first walked in, I was taken aback: I had never seen a room full of curly headed women before. It was like visiting a homeland for curly hair!

As a result, my relationship with my hair is now as easy as it should be. There's lots of real, unavoidable suffering in the world, and none of it should be about the texture of your hair!

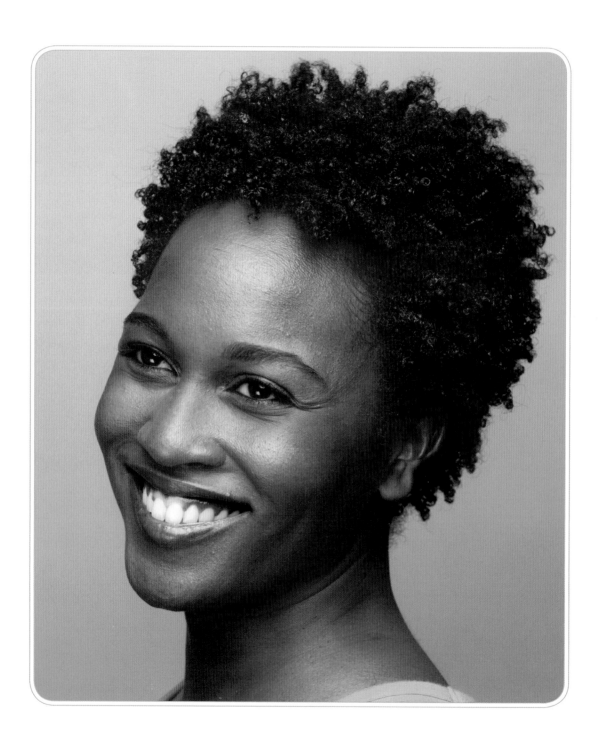

multi-curl-tural hair

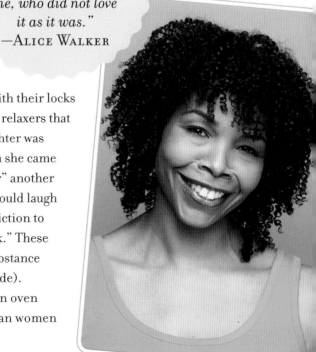

> *"Eventually I knew what hair wanted; it wanted to be itself . . . to be left alone by anyone, including me, who did not love it as it was."*
> —ALICE WALKER

I remember hearing actor Chris Rock talk about the impetus for his movie *Good Hair*, a documentary exploring African American women's relationship with their locks and the $9 billion industry of weaves, wigs, and relaxers that it has spawned. The idea hit him when his daughter was raving about her friend's hair one day and when she came home crying because she didn't have "good hair" another day. When I saw the movie, I didn't know if I should laugh or cry when several women described their addiction to chemical relaxers as "being on the creamy crack." These relaxers are made of lye, a corrosive alkaline substance (either sodium hydroxide or potassium hydroxide).

Besides straightening hair, lye is used as an oven cleaner and drain opener! But African American women are not alone in their struggles with their hair. We are a multicultural world. It's not a one-size-fits-all globe anymore, especially regarding hair. We have many multi-curl-tural clients at Devachan Salon, so I decided to hand over this chapter to a convert and expert on the subject, Vida Vladirm, of Devachan.

Vida's Advice for Multi-curl-tural Hair

Though there are exceptions, many ethnic groups have very curly hair. Some of these include Latin Americans, African Americans, Jews, and Italians, but the list goes on and on. Then there are those of us of mixed nationalities who have multitextured hair. But no matter what ethnicity you are, you don't have to live with dull, dry, brittle locks. What you have can be changed, perhaps not overnight but through persistence. If you want to be free of what I call modern-day slavery to your hair, a lot of patience and large amounts of moisturizing conditioners are key.

Traditionally, we multicultural women have used products that contain petroleum, silicone, waxes, and dry oils, believing that they will control, protect, and hydrate their hair. But rather than being absorbed and providing moisture, these products sit on the hair's surface, repelling water like a duck's feathers and attracting dirt. No wonder our hair looks dull and lifeless!

When it's time for our weekly washing, the first rinse of water that goes down the drain is mucky and brown. It sounds gross, but that's the dirt that's been sitting in the hair for a week finally getting flushed out. Typically we cleanse again and apply conditioner, which isn't on the hair long enough to offer much benefit, especially when the hair has been trapped under heavy petroleum and waxes for a week. Then we reapply those same moisture-robbing products, so the hair never gets the hydration it really needs and deserves. And therein lies (or should I say lyes) the problem.

All curls need moisture, but multicultural curls are *desperately begging* for hydration, especially those curls that are smaller and tighter. And though multicultural hair can appear thick, each strand is actually very fine and weak, so all this gunk we put on our hair and stuff we do to straighten it takes a toll on our hair, not to mention our wallet. I know this all too well because it's exactly what I did—for decades.

When I was growing up, my hair was braided into two little ponytails or put in Shirley Temple sausage curls at the salon.

Other times, both as a little girl and an adult, I had my hair straightened with a hot comb or flat iron, which more than once was too hot and singed

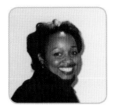

Vida with relaxed hair.

my hair off and caused burns on my scalp, forehead, ears, and neck. I also used to abuse my curls when sleeping by putting in nearly fifty plastic perming rods, with the hope that they would tame and smooth my hair. They were uncomfortable, but my hair was more important than sleeping well. Then one day I realized that it was crazy— as well as hypocritical—for me to tell my clients at the salon to love their curly hair while I relaxed and disguised mine.

Yes, I decided it was time to let my hair be. I didn't make any big commitments and I always kept a bottle of relaxer in my fridge at home, just

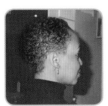

Vida goes natural.

in case. I went cold turkey. Now, some people prefer to go curly more gradually by softening their hair first with what they believe are gentle relaxers. But remember that by doing so, your curls won't emerge as quickly, if at all, or will be lethargic. That said, I know you need to find your own comfort level.

At first, I'd braid my hair or do a two-strand twist, let it dry, and then unravel it. But my hair didn't grow very much and I didn't see many curls.

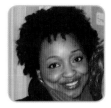

Vida in transition.

Finally, I had to admit that I really needed to leave my hair alone once and for all. So I started following the routine for multi-curl-tural hair (described in detail, pages 65–69): I gave up shampoo and slathered my dry hair with a botanical conditioner, starting at the ends and working it throughout my whole head of hair. Often, I'd keep the conditioner in my hair for an entire weekend.

My hair began to grow faster than I imagined it could. The first section of curls cropped up in the back of my head; the last in the front and on top, which makes sense since those are the areas most exposed to environmental damage. Soon my hair was below my bra strap. Years ago, if you'd told me that I'd have the curls I do today, I would have said you were crazy, thinking "other people's hair may grow like that, but my hair doesn't." But it did. And so can yours. **Note:** For more tips on going natural, see chapter 7, Curlies Coming Out of the Closet.

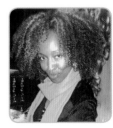

Vida's amazing curls today.

So if you're ready to put down the chemicals, relaxers, and hot combs and go natural, understand that your curls are not going to happen overnight, *but they will come*. However, they're not going to reach their full potential until the products full of petroleum, waxes, and silicones are no longer clinging to your strands. Keeping hair in optimum condition during the growing-out phase is paramount, because you want the new growth to be healthy. Coconut oils, shea butter, jojoba oil, and TLCurl are all key moisturizers to use during this phase and in the future to keep your hair hydrated. Your hair will start to lie a little softer once it's no longer being abused.

Begin by following the cleansing and styling routines for fractal and zigzag curls, on the next page. At first you will need to

curl confession

Stephanie Trusty *bookkeeper and staff accountant*

Starting around the age of nine, my sister would straighten my tight, kinky hair with a hot comb heated on the stove using either lard or very thick hair pomade. The whole house would smell like something was burning. After that, I graduated to permanent relaxers, but that thinned out my hair around the edges and in other spots.

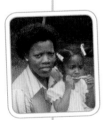

Then I went natural, but couldn't stand it, so I tried getting my hair hot-combed at a salon. The tips of my ears got burnt and smoke filled up the place with such heat that I could hardly stand it—all just to get my hair straight! I tried to sleep with rollers in my hair but it was torture. The final straw happened when a beautician put a softener in my hair that left my hair smelling like rotten fish for a month despite many, many washings.

Finally, I was tired and frustrated by my quest to find the "perfect solution." My hair wanted to be curly. I had to stop fighting it, and I cut my hair really short. I wondered if my hair made me look unattractive to men. (I know it shouldn't have mattered, but it did.) So it meant a lot to me when my oldest brother, whose opinion I highly value, told me how great it looked. Many of my friends say they wish they could just let their hair go, but they think their husbands won't like it. My advice? Give it a try! It is so liberating not to have to spend the time and money in salons and on products trying to figure out how to tame my hair. It took a while, but I finally learned that what my hair really wanted was for me to let it be its kinky, curly self.

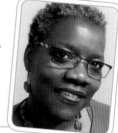

Afro-zen

Growing out hair treated by relaxers can be a pain, but relax (pun intended). Be Zen and adventurous with it. Some creative ideas to help you through this awkward phase include:

■ Hats, headbands, clips, and other hair adornments can be helpful enhancements.

■ Go for a Billie Holiday jazz singer look that is sleek, slicked back, and anchored with clips, a flower, or brooch at the side.

■ The Afraux-hawk is so popular in an updo shape and can be very flattering with all hair types and face shapes. Simply slick or braid back the sides and allow the top center to be freestanding and natural.

■ The "twist and out" is a great day-to-evening look. Twist or braid locks when wet for daytime, so they set the hair but still look stylish. Then at night, unleash them by gently opening them apart and shaking out your curls so they're voluminous and sexy.

■ Hairpieces can be playful, when clipped in temporarily for a stylish look.

use a sulfate-free cleanser or botanical conditioner several times a week to really release all the waxy product from your hair. I also recommend that you condition your hair nightly as I did. Also, leaving some, maybe all, of the conditioner in your hair when you shower can be a good styling foundation. If you have flyaways, put some gel in your hands and glide it over your wet hair. The next day, your hair will probably still look great and the bathroom steam will reactivate your curl product from the day before.

DAILY ROUTINE FOR

FRACTAL AND ZIGZAG CURLS

■ **Cleansing/conditioning and styling time:** 10 to 15 minutes. This time will decrease when hydration has become your hair's way of life.

Fractal and zigzag curls are the tiniest, driest, and densest of any hair type. Because of their nonporous nature, a lot of products don't penetrate the hair shaft, which is why you may have tried unsuccessfully to hydrate your hair in the past. You know by now that sulfate-filled products are bad for curls, and for fractals and zigzags they're a disaster. Just one dose of shampoo takes gallons of water to rinse and it never comes out completely. For these curl types to absorb maximum moisture, they need to be hydrated *before* you get in the shower. A precleanse acts as a wetting agent for these hard-to-saturate fractals and zigzags, making the conditioning process more effective. This method is also great for cleansing dreadlocks, weaves, or extensions.

coloring multi-curl-tural curls

Though you can color your curly hair (I use a lightener on mine), you have to be careful. Hair color chemicals can dehydrate your already parched curls. Just make sure you are conditioning and deep conditioning on a regular basis, in order to put back the moisture that's depleted when hair coloring products are used. And remember: No shampoo! Ever!

Cleansing and Conditioning

1 Before getting in the shower, pour a shallow palmful of sulfate-free cleanser or botanical conditioner into one hand, then rub your hands together. (If you're not sure whether to use cleanser or conditioner, go with the latter because it is more hydrating.) Smooth the cleanser or conditioner over the entire surface of the hair's canopy, using a downward motion. This precleanse acts as a wetting agent to

make the cleansing and conditioning process more effective. (It saves water, too.)

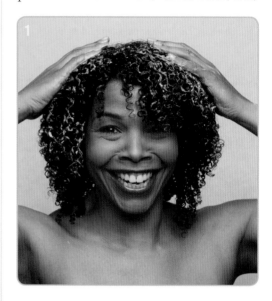

2 Turn on the shower and stand under the water stream to wet your hair thoroughly.

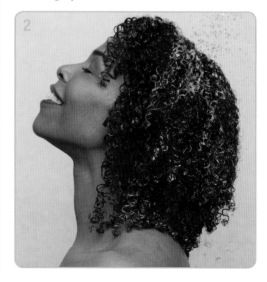

3 Cup one hand, apply a sulfate-free cleanser or botanical conditioner along your fingertips and distribute to the fingertips of your other hand. Starting at the temples, place your fingertips on your scalp and use a firm, circular massaging motion to rub gently down the sides of your head. Move to the top of your head, massaging gently toward the crown; then move to the back of the head, ending at the nape of the neck.

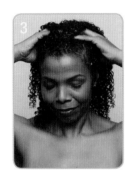

4 Rinse your hair thoroughly.

5 Take a generous palmful of botanical conditioner and apply it throughout the landscape of the hair, so no curl is left behind. Again, err on the side of more rather than less for this hair type. Your hair should have as much viscosity as a jellyfish in water. Cleanse or shave another body part while you let the conditioner soak into your curls.

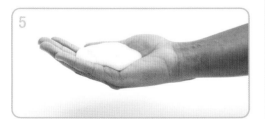

6 Gently comb your fingertips through your hair from underneath, removing knots and loose hairs that have naturally gathered. Don't worry if hairs come out; it's normal to lose about a hundred hairs a day. Continue to comb conditioner through the hairs' terrain.

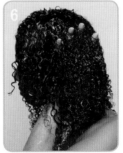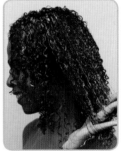

7 Do not rinse out the conditioner, or at the most, splash a handful or two of water on the surface of the hair to help disperse the conditioner through the landscape of the hair. Turn off the water, but stay in the shower. Tilt your head to one side and use your hands to squeeze-quench your hair up toward the scalp so a milky residue seeps through your fingers. (Because of the density and dryness of this curl type, the hair may not drip at all.)

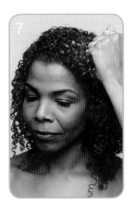

Hair ex-Tensions

I'm not a big fan of braiding multicultural hair because often it is pulled and tugged so tightly at the scalp that the hairline begins to recede. Unfortunately, once the hair recedes it doesn't grow back. I'm also not big on hair extensions. I've seen women who have had them in for years and years, and underneath the artificial strands, their own hair has receded so much that the extension is hanging barely by a thread of real hair.

Styling

1 After you step out of the shower, let the conditioner seep in for two to three minutes as you dry the rest of your body.

2 If you are not looking for more height or width, do not tilt your head forward. Instead, look up to the ceiling and sway your hair back and forth to allow it to fall into its natural place. Take a generous palmful of gel and rub it onto both hands. Tilt your head to the right, and evenly distribute gel into the hair as you scrunch-squeeze hair gently up toward the scalp. Tilt head to the left and do the same scrunch-squeeze motion.

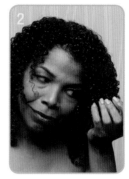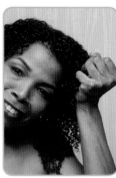

3 Rub another shallow palmful of gel between your hands and lightly graze it downward over the entire canopy of the hair. Fractal and zigzag curls can soak in all the moisturizing product you give them.

4 If you *do* want hair to have more height or width, at Step 2 tilt your head over and apply gel with both hands as you scrunch-squeeze hair gently up toward the scalp. Then scrunch gel throughout the canopy of the hair.

5 With your head still tilted over, place your hands lightly on your scalp and use your fingertips to gently shuffle your hair at the roots, which will give it some lift. With your hands still on your scalp, stand upright and lift your hands off your head without raking your fingers through your hair. If you want more lift, place clips at the roots (see page 41).

curl confession

Christine Carter Lynch *administrator for a financial firm*

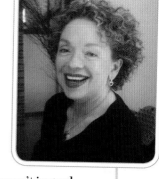

Though I had what's considered "good hair" in African American culture, it was still hard to manage as a child. All my girlfriends had cute little bobs, but if my hair was down it just looked wild. To tame it, my mom would brush it every morning (the pain from that was excruciating) and braid it. A few times I had my hair chemically straightened, and other times I used rollers and sat under a dryer to smooth it. When I started working on Wall Street, I would get my hair professionally blow-dried every week and wouldn't wash it until the next week. (My hairdresser used to say that he developed his muscles from blowing

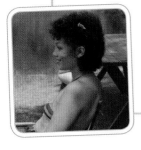

out my hair because it was so much work.)

Then I ran into two friends who had let their hair go curly and they looked gorgeous, so I decided to do the same. My hair wasn't in good condition at first, but I was patient and let it grow. It's so easy for your hair, especially African American hair, to enslave you, but obsessing over it isn't a good use of energy. If you just let it do what it wants to do and keep it healthy, you're going to look good. I am at a really good place in my life right now and I know embracing my hair has helped.

6 It's best to let your hair air dry, because your curls are fragile and heat can sometimes evaporate the gel. But if you don't have time, dry it with a diffuser (see page 55), hooded dryer (they're surprisingly inexpensive and portable), or if you're on the go, put your heater on in the car.

"It has been ten years since I last combed my hair! Family and friends are sometimes scandalized! I am amused by their reactions. During those ten years, they have poured gallons of possibly carcinogenic relaxer chemicals on themselves, and their once proud crinkled or kinky hair has been forced to lie flat as a slab over a grave. I understand this, I did this same thing to myself."
—ALICE WALKER

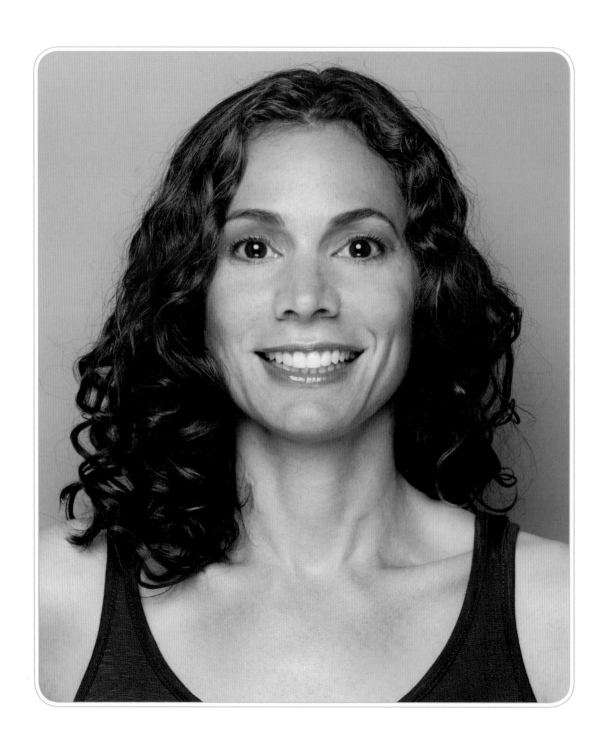

CHAPTER 7

relax? don't do it

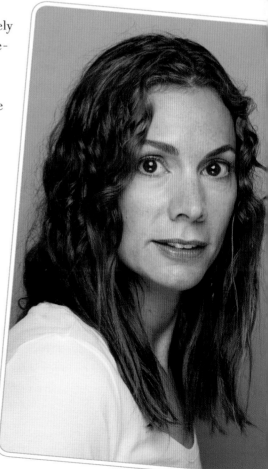

Chemical straightening treatments were extremely popular about six or seven years ago when bone-straight hair was all the rage. Called Japanese straightening, thermal reconditioning, or Brazilian Keratin Treatment, among other names, these treatments use extremely strong chemicals and a special flat iron to alter the internal structure of the hair so that its curly bonds are changed to straight ones. It sounds simple, but it's not. First of all, these treatments are time consuming, taking six to eight hours the first time you get it done and four to six hours to get your roots touched up. It also costs from $300 to $1,000 per treatment. But the worst part is that the treatments' harsh chemicals can weaken the hair, causing split ends and breakage at the roots. This breakage leaves a halo of floating strands on top of your head—not a good look.

Chemical straightening is permanent, so the only way to return to your curly roots is to wait for your hair to grow out, and that can take months or even years. (Some salons claim that their Brazilian straightening treatment is not permanent but wears off over the course of a few months. However, that's not always the case.) Plus, the results that you've paid so much time and money for aren't always pretty. I often hear chemically straightened girls, even those who like their smoother strands, complain that they can wear only one hairstyle that is pin-straight and flat against the head. Still, many are willing to be stuck with that look rather than the curly hair they don't know how to manage. Often, you can't color hair if you straighten it with one of these treatments, because the combination of chemicals can break your strands. Unfortunately, salons that tout these treatments and their unrealistic expectations don't prepare you for the fallout.

Worse yet, these treatments may not be good for your health. An article in *Allure* magazine, "Scared Straight," cautioned readers about the dangers of the popular Brazilian straightening treatment, and described the frightening lengths women will go to for sleek hair. The details in the article gave me chills: Two women and their hairstylist wear

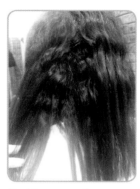

Healthy new curls sprout beneath the straightened hair.

$700 military-grade rubber gas masks to keep from smelling the chemicals' potent, unhealthy fumes. One of the known ingredients in some straightening is formaldehyde, which has been classified as a human carcinogen by the International Agency for Research on Cancer, part of the World Health Organization.

Many salons took the Brazilian straightening treatment off their menus soon after this story ran or say they use a formaldehyde-free version of it, but it's hard to know exactly what they're putting on your hair, so you are straightening at your own risk.

Now, if you're a curly girl who has been having her hair chemically straightened but wants to return to her curly roots, welcome back! Don't worry, your curls will be forgiving no matter how badly you've treated them. I'll be honest, though, growing out chemically straightened hair isn't easy. But when you're ready, you are ready! And it *is* worth it. Now, your hair may not feel or look right when you first start to grow it out. As the healthy, new curls sprout, they act like little springs and push out the straightened hair. The result is two personalities of hair on your head: the regrowth of your natural, curly texture at the top and your chemically straightened hair at the bottom. You can cut your hair starting where the new curls end and the straight hair begins, but most closeted curly girls won't do this. Or you can wait for your hair to grow and for your curls to take over. How long this takes depends on the rate your hair grows and your curls' spring factor. It will take time, patience, and absolute willpower. But you can do it! While your curls grow in, here are a few things you can do:

■ Toss out every bottle of shampoo. As you know by now, most shampoos contain harsh detergents that further dry out hair that's parched and damaged from chemical treatments, and it never rinses out completely. Though conditioner can soften and smooth hair, even the most superior product won't be able to repair overwashed and exhausted hair cuticle.

■ Start hydrating your hair with daily conditioning treatments ASAP. Your poor hair needs superhydration to repair itself from the straightening chemicals and to make sure the new curly growth is its healthiest. If you see a halo of frizz as your curls grow in, it just means that your hair hasn't been hydrated enough. Keep it at bay by using conditioner, conditioner, and more conditioner.

■ Say good-bye to your brush. The act of brushing or combing the hair interferes with your curls' formation, causing dispersed curls—otherwise known as frizz! Even when your hair is more straight than curly, you should get out of the brushing habit. Instead, use your fingers to comb through the hair—and then *only* while it's wet and drenched with conditioner.

■ Get your hair trimmed often. Most curly girls don't want to cut off all their straight hair, but you do need regular trims to "oxygenize" the hair. This means you refresh and aerate the hair so it can take in more oxygen and moisture, which helps those curly strands grow in faster.

■ Experiment with ways to style your hair while it's growing out. Use leave-in conditioner and slick your hair back in a classic knot at the back of the head or off to the side. Try some of the updos in chapter 15, page 157; wear bandannas or hats. Just make sure you don't pull your hair back too tightly or you'll cause your hairline to recede. And always use ponytail holders without clasps that can cut through the hair.

■ You can use clips to curl the straightened hair to match your curl pattern (see Making Waves sidebar, right, for details). But never use curling irons and, even worse, never perm the straight ends to match your curly roots, because the hair can break off. Setbacks set you back!

■ Eat a healthy diet that helps hair grow (see chapter 3, page 29, for tips).

■ Don't be tempted to blow-fry or flat iron your roots to match your straight ends.

Remember that straightening your curls is temporary—lasting only until your next shower or the next time it rains. Loving your curls and living with them is permanent! Also, those new roots are healthy, unprocessed hair and will eventually be your happy ends, so baby them. You want to nurture your curls, because soon you'll have gorgeous, healthy hair without much effort.

■ To stay motivated, visualize how your curls will look in a few months.

curl confession

Maria Barrios *teacher*

I went to the salon for a basic blow-out, but the stylist put a permanent relaxer on my curls without telling me! The shampoo, conditioning, and blow-out had taken a long time, but I thought that was because my hair was so thick. It wasn't until I washed my hair that I realized it wasn't curly anymore. My mother, who's a hairdresser, took one look and knew immediately what had happened. Still, I couldn't believe that a hair stylist would relax someone's hair without discussing it first!

Then, when I went to get highlights, my hair broke off. First my curls had been straightened and now they were falling out! I was devastated. My hair had been one of my best attributes. I had to dye it pitch black (which looked bad with my very pale skin) so that the damage was less noticeable. For the next year and a half, I took really good care of my hair so that the curls growing in would be in good condition. Now it's almost grown out, but I'll never trust just anyone with my hair again!

Making waves

If your hair is naturally straight or if you are growing out straightened hair and have two hair types on your head, this method will help merge your two hair personalities into one.

1. Use the cleansing routine for wavy and s'wavy hair (see chapter 5, page 52).

2. Tilt your head forward and cup the hair loosely in a paper towel, microfiber towel, or an old cotton T-shirt. Scrunch-squeeze as much water out of your hair as possible.

3. With your head still tilted, evenly distribute a palmful of gel throughout your hair with both hands, using the same scrunch-squeeze moation you did with the towel. You will start to see some wave formation in your hair.

4. Keeping your head tilted, use a blow-dryer (preferably an ionic one) with a diffuser on a low to medium heat setting until your hair is almost dry.

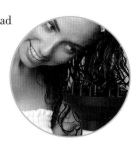

5. Then stand upright and wrap sections of your hair tightly around your fingers, starting at the knuckle and going toward the fingertip. For tighter curls, use your pinky, and for slightly bigger waves, use two or three fingers. With different sections of hair, choose different widths, which will make the waves appear more natural.

6. Spray a clip with spray gel, and place the clip in the curl perpendicular to the scalp. This adds lift and softens a strong part. Old-fashioned hairnets work wonders in keeping hair in a holding pattern while you've got clips in your hair.

7. Leave clips in longer if your hair is quite straight or you want more defined waves; leave them in for a shorter time for looser waves. Gently remove the clips by holding the curl with one hand and opening the clip with the other.

8. Lean over and tilt your head forward, place your splayed fingers lightly on your scalp, and gently shuffle the hair at the roots. Stand upright and lift the hands away from your scalp without raking your fingers through your hair.

9. Once hair is dry, loosen the gel cast by gently scrunching upward with your fingers in the same way you applied the gel. Then mist with spray gel (see page 80 for recipe).

10. For the Rita Hayworth look, hold your head upright and gently finger comb through your hair to fuse the waves together.

curl confession

Michele Bender *coauthor,* Curly Girl

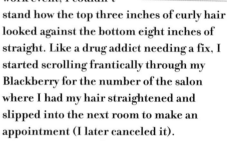

Though I'm a naturally curly girl, I was in total denial for six years. The first time I got my hair chemically straightened, the stylist asked, "Are you sure you're ready for poker-straight strands?" Truth be told, I didn't care if I looked like Marcia Brady. I couldn't stand another day of frizz and as the mother of a one-year-old, I had no time to spend on my curls. Once he was done, I loved the results—finally, I had shiny, soft strands that blew in the wind and didn't frizz.

Cut to six years later. It was time to get my hair straightened again, but I just couldn't do it. First, I was tired of the flat, plastered-to-my-head look that chemically straightened hair often has. Second, I hated the feeling that the moment I stepped out of the salon, the curly hair time clock was ticking. And, third, I noticed some gray and knew that coloring *and* straightening was too much for my hair to handle. Most important, I was working with Lorraine on this book, and I had interviewed so many women who grew up hating their curls like I did but had learned to treat them right and now actually loved their hair. Too bad, that now that I knew how to make my curls look great, I didn't have them anymore.

So I set out on a journey to go curly. I knew it wouldn't be easy and that I'd have to spend at least a year or more with two textures of hair on my head. One time before an important work event, I couldn't stand how the top three inches of curly hair looked against the bottom eight inches of straight. Like a drug addict needing a fix, I started scrolling frantically through my Blackberry for the number of the salon where I had my hair straightened and slipped into the next room to make an appointment (I later canceled it).

During most of that year, I religiously conditioned my hair in the shower, and then at night I'd slather more conditioner on my dry hair and sleep on a satin pillow, knowing my curls were coated in hydration. I became obsessed with noticing curly hair—on the subway, at coffee shops, at my kids' school—and when gazing into the bathroom mirror. I started a blog on Naturallycurly.com, and was amazed at how much I had to say about my hair.

There were many months when my hair looked like a bowl of mixed pasta: The top looked like elbow macaroni; the bottom, angel hair pasta; and underneath, rotini. I was shocked that I wasn't even tempted to blow-dry my hair. I figured that if I was going for the curl, I wanted to give those virgin hairs a fighting chance and let them be. Almost two years later, I finally have most of my curls back. And I promise to spend the rest of my life giving them the respect they deserve!

CHAPTER 8

products and homemade recipes

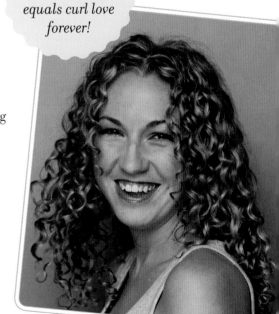

Curl knowledge and wisdom equals curl love forever!

If you're like most curly girls, you've spent a lot of time and money searching for the product that is *the one*. You imagined that, like a knight in shining armor, it would rescue your curls from frizz, flyaways, and dryness. It's this continual search for frizz-free locks and our severely misunderstood hair type that keeps the big beauty companies in big business. When I peruse the aisles of beauty supply stores, I'm amazed at the language used to describe products that claim to be made for us curlies, such as "taming," "controlling," "sealing," and "flattening."

These words are chosen to intimidate us and make us feel less than OK, again and again and again. Faced with all this jargon, what's a curly girl to do? Don't be fooled by the hype! Be an educated curly consumer. Know what you're looking for in a product and learn how to read a label.

Ingredients at the beginning of the list are the highest amounts in the product; ingredients toward the end of the list are included in smaller amounts, and ones near the very end are in such small amounts as to be meaningless.

THE GOOD, THE BAD, AND THE BUBBLY

The array of shampoos, conditioners, and styling products that fill store shelves is dizzying and overwhelming. But it doesn't have to be. What follows is a guide to finding the right products to keep your curls looking their best.

curl confession

Robin Berger *attorney*

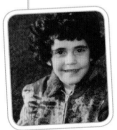

As a child, I could never find anyone who knew how to cut my thick, curly hair (or knew what to do with it). When I got older and tried to grow it long, my curls would grow out instead of down, so I looked like Bozo the Clown. I spent hundreds and hundreds of dollars on products and tried salons that claimed to specialize in curls, but they were terrible. One left my hair looking like an oil slick, and suggested that I apply a product that actually removed my nail polish every time I used it. I wondered, if it's doing that to my polish, what's it doing to my hair?

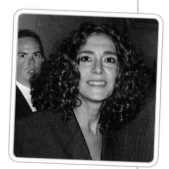

Then I finally found a salon where they knew how to cut my curls. My first haircut felt like the greatest thing that had ever happened to me. Afterward, my social life picked up like you wouldn't believe. My hair never looks bad (even at its worst, it looks better than it did when I was growing up), and I'm constantly stopped on the street and asked about my hair. My only regret is that I didn't realize I had this beautiful hair earlier in my life.

THE GOOD, THE BAD, AND THE BUBBLY

Cleansers

Look for **sulfate-free** products only. Detergents frequently found in shampoo are sulfates such as sodium lauryl sulfate (the harshest), ammonium laureth sulfate (also harsh), and sodium laureth sulfate (harsh). Always check the ingredients list on the product to make sure none of these detergents are included.

Conditioners

Look for a **botanical conditioner.** Botanicals should contain high concentrations of plant-based ingredients such as mint, lemongrass, and rosemary. They will help maintain a photoprotective shield around hair shafts. And many botanicals offer specific benefits to curly hair, like adding moisture. Make sure that the plants used in the product are listed in the first half of the ingredients list; otherwise the amount is too negligible to be helpful to your hair.

Look for a conditioner that contains:

▥ **Emollients** soften hair and reduce frizz by smoothing the cuticle. There are hundreds of emollients, but some good ones for curly hair include shea butter, vegetable oils, olive oil, walnut oil, jojoba oil, cetyl esters, and wheat germ.

▥ **Humectants** absorb water from the atmosphere and hang on to it. They're absolutely crucial in a conditioner for curly hair. Some to look for include panthenol, vegetable glycerin, and sorbitol.

▥ **Moisturizers** add softness and control to curly hair. Look for amino acids, aloe vera, olive oil, balm mint extracts, and propylene glycol.

Steer clear of products that contain:

▥ **Silicone.** This synthetic material is the active ingredient in many conditioners and 99 percent of shine products. Often used in manufacturing rubber, plastics, and polishes, it's actually made to repel water and isn't biodegradable. So any product with silicone in it will act as a seal around the cuticle, preventing the absorption of moisture. Silicone can also weigh down your curls, preventing their natural shape from emerging.

Gels

When shopping for gel, do the skin test. Apply a little bit to your hands and rub them together. If it feels sticky on your skin, it will probably feel sticky on your hair. Also avoid products that say they are "styling creams" or "waxes." These make hair crispy, like Ramen noodles (not a good look!).

Also, steer clear of gel that contains:

▧ **Alcohol.** Curls should be seen and not heard, and alcohols in gels can cause hair sound effects. The right gel will leave your hair frizz-free and touchable, and all you'll hear is how curlicious you look! Certain alcohols, like cetyl alcohol, are okay if they're in a cleanser, but those used in gels can be extremely drying for hair and cause frizz. Plus, unlike cleansers, which get rinsed out quickly, gel lives in a curly girl's locks for a day or more. If the gel contains alcohol, it will spend those days sucking up your strands' moisture and will prevent new hydration from getting in.

▧ **Silicone.** You don't want silicone in your gel for the same reasons you don't want it in your conditioner. It repels water, preventing the hair from absorbing the moisture it needs. And a gel is on the hair longer than any other product.

▧ **Parabens.** One of the most widely used preservatives added to cosmetics (as well as foods and drugs) to ward off the growth of bacteria. Those you'll typically find in an ingredients list include methylparaben, propylparaben, and butylparaben. In recent years, they've become controversial as experts question whether they are safe. (Some say they may be linked to cancer.)

▧ **Phthalates.** Used in plastics for longevity; many are being phased out because of health concerns.

Make a spray gel

Spray styling gels are basically diluted versions of gels. They're especially good on loose, wavy curls because the mist gets lightly distributed through the hair without weighing it down. They're also a wonderful way to refresh all hair types during the day. You can buy one or make your own spray gel by combining ½ cup gel with 1 cup boiled water. Allow the mixture to cool, then pour it into a spray bottle. If you think your hair needs a stronger hold, experiment by gradually adding more gel to the mixture until you achieve the consistency that works best for your curls.

HERBAL ABUSE

Many products claim to be "natural," "organic," "herbal," or full of "botanical ingredients"—even those you buy at well-known stores. But what do those words really mean as applied to beauty products? Not very much. The claims are not regulated, so any company can add those words to their labels and many of them do, touting their organic or natural status to make you think you're "going green." (It's called "greenwashing.")

The only way to know if a product is organic is if you see the USDA Organic seal, which means that 95 percent of the ingredients in the product are organic. If the product says "Made with certified organic ingredients," this means 70 to 95 percent of its ingredients are organic. In some cases, it also means it should be in the refrigerator. Yet, just because a product says that it's natural or organic doesn't mean it's good for your curly hair! Again, check the ingredients list on the bottle against the lists on pages 79–80 and make sure it doesn't contain any of the ingredients we say you should avoid.

curl confession

Julie Weiss *art director*, Vanity Fair

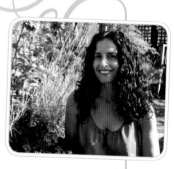

The secret—and most essential—ingredient for our hair's health and happiness is the simplest thing in the world: water. It's a natural tonic. Just like in the garden, where plants need water to come alive and grow, so does our curly hair. Whenever I feel that my hair is wilting or losing its shine, I wet it and it immediately comes back to life. The curls form again and look alive. It's similar to how tired, wilted lettuce will come back to life when placed in a bowl of cool water.

Thinking about how water affects our hair, I am reminded of how I loved to water gardens when I was a little girl. Whenever our family would go to friends or relatives' houses with a garden, I would always ask if I could water it. I didn't care if it was just a few plants in front of an apartment building, I loved the feeling of helping these plants come to life. Immediately, their colors were brighter, the greens looked greener, and the soil looked deep and rich instead of dry. I found it so relaxing and meditative. Everyone knows that water can be healing for people and for plants, flowers, and trees. It can also do the same for our curly hair.

HOMEMADE RECIPES

POETRY IN POTIONS

The only way to be totally sure that a product includes ingredients that are good for your curls is to make your own. This is something I love to do. On weekends with friends, we experiment and concoct new lotions 'n' potions. The following are our tried-and-true tested favorites:

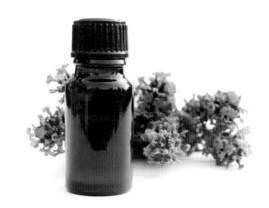

DEEP-PACK CHAKRA

This calming protein pack will soften your hair and create beautiful curls while soothing your spirit. The amount of water you use to make the protein rinse varies depending on the length and thickness of your hair: Use 1 cup water for short, thinner hair, or 2 cups water for long, thick hair. Powdered egg, jojoba oil, and verbena essence can be found at most health food stores.

> *1 tablespoon powdered egg*
> *1 tablespoon powdered milk*
> *1/2 teaspoon honey, combined with a few drops of hot water to soften*
> *2 tablespoons olive oil or jojoba oil*
> *1 or 2 cups pasta water (for added nutrients), or plain boiled water*
> *1 or 2 drops verbena essence, or your preferred fragrant oil*

1. Combine the powdered egg, powdered milk, softened honey, and olive oil to form a smooth paste.
2. Add the water and the herbal essence, and stir to combine.
3. Pour the entire mixture over well-rinsed hair.
4. Wrap your hair with clear plastic wrap, making a turban, and allow the protein rinse to penetrate the hair for 1 hour or more.
5. Rinse well. Cleanse and/or condition, then style.

LAVENDER-IT-WITH-LOVE SPRAY

Lavender has cleansing properties, so this spray can cleanse and deodorize the hair and scalp. (The word *lavender* comes from the French word *laver*, which means to clean or wash.) It not only makes your hair smell like a Provençal lavender field, but it's also indispensable for cleansing and reviving your curls. Make it in large quantities, and then keep some in a big spray bottle in your shower and in smaller travel-sized bottles in your purse, desk, and car for spritz on the go. Spray bottles are available at most drugstores and essential oils are available at most health food stores.

> *2 quarts water*
> *5 drops pure (not synthetic) lavender essential oil*

1. Fill a large pot with the water.
2. Cover the pot, bring the water to a boil on high heat, then turn the heat down to low and simmer for 1 hour to get rid of impurities. (Check occasionally to make sure the water isn't boiling away.)
3. Remove the water from the heat, add the lavender oil, stir to blend, and replace the lid.
4. Let the lavender water steep until cool, then pour it into spray bottles.
5. Store extra lavender spray in a cool place.

MULTITASK WITH lavender spray

Lavender spray makes a wonderful gift for friends, whether they are curly girls or not. Once you get hooked on the spray, you'll find lots of other uses for it. Some of my clients have told me that their husbands sprayed it on them in the delivery room, because lavender is known to have a calming effect. You can also:

■ Use it as a room and car deodorizer.

■ Spray it on bed linens to help you drift off to sleep.

■ Spray it on clothes in the dryer to add a fresh scent.

■ Use it to refresh your hair, face, and clothes after cooking or barbecuing.

■ Keep it in your air travel bag so you can spritz on the plane.

SCRUB-ME-THE-RIGHT-WAY EXFOLIATING CLEANSER

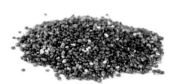

We know that exfoliating is good for improving the condition of your skin. Since your scalp is also skin, an exfoliating treatment once a week will slough off dead skin cells or conditioner buildup, and relieve any itchiness. But don't confuse dandruff with dry scalp. Or worse, don't fall off the no-poo wagon and use a dandruff shampoo that contains harsh detergents. Instead, try this scrub when your scalp feels drier than usual, like during the winter months. Quinoa is a grain available at health food stores.

1 tablespoon brown sugar or uncooked quinoa
3 tablespoons conditioner

1. Mix together the brown sugar or quinoa and the conditioner, and stir to create a thick paste.
2. Wet your hair in the shower, then put the paste on your fingertips. Starting at the nape of your neck and moving upward, gently massage the paste on your scalp in a circular motion. Linger on any spots that seem tense or itchy.
3. Rinse your hair thoroughly, then condition and style.

Makes scalp scrub for 1 session

WRAPUNZEL

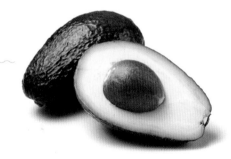

Inspired by the Mayans, this rich avocado hair treat will nourish and moisturize dry ends. Jojoba oil and agave can be found at most health food stores.

1 ripe avocado, peeled and cored
3 to 4 teaspoons honey or agave syrup
8 to 10 drops olive oil or jojoba oil

1. Put the avocado, honey, and oil in a blender. Blend briefly until combined.
2. Apply the avocado mixture to your wet hair, especially targeting the ends.
3. Wrap your hair with clear plastic wrap or a towel, making a turban. Leave on for 20 to 30 minutes.
4. Rinse your hair thoroughly, cleanse and/or condition, then style.

LEMON AID

This moisturizing and neutralizing tonic will remove chlorine and protect hair in hard water regions. It's especially good for very dry or damaged locks.

Combine the juice of 1 large lemon with your usual amount of conditioner. Apply the lemon-conditioner mixture to wet hair, then rinse.

COOL CURLS are HOT!

One thing that really helps frizz-prone hair during warm weather months is to keep all your gel and styling products in the fridge. (If you forget to do this, stick them in the freezer for about 10 minutes before using.) The cold closes the cuticle of your hair shafts, leaving you frizz-free! In the winter, do the opposite: Warm your conditioner in the microwave for a minute or two, apply your gel or style product, and wrap your head with a warm towel. Leave on for half an hour.

SWIM-IN-LOVE

Here's a fabulous trick for protecting your hair when swimming in a pool: In addition to applying conditioner, pick up one of those sleek-looking oil spray misters at any housewares store. Fill it with olive oil and a few drops of your favorite herbal essence. Spritz the fragrant oil on your hair before jumping into the pool or spritz the lining of a bathing cap before putting it on your head. The oil will help protect your hair from the damaging chlorinated water.

ALOE, GOOD-BYE

Aloe vera is a completely natural hydrating and conditioning substance that is therapeutic for your scalp. It's also great to use on your hair after you've been to the beach or before and after hair coloring treatments. Be sure to get the edible type of aloe vera gel (the kind that has to be refrigerated after opening), which can be found at health food stores.

After you've cleansed and rinsed your hair with warm water, apply a generous amount of aloe vera gel to your scalp. Massage the scalp gently for several minutes. Rinse your hair, and then condition it as usual. Or massage the gel into your dry scalp and leave it overnight.

You can also leave aloe vera gel in your hair as an alternative for styling gel: Just add 3 drops of your favorite herbal essence oil to a 3-ounce bottle of aloe vera, and scrunch it into your hair.

TLC (TENDER LOVING CURLS)

This revitalizing oil treatment will nourish the ends of your hair. It's especially useful in winter, when your ends are in constant friction with wool and other heavy fabrics. The amount of oil you use depends on the length and thickness of your hair. You can add one or more essential oils found at most health food stores.

1 to 3 teaspoons olive oil, jojoba oil, or shea butter
2 to 4 drops pure essential oil, like lavender, verbena, or vanilla

1. Combine the olive oil and the essential oil, and apply it to the ends of your hair.
2. Wrap your hair with clear plastic wrap, like a turban, and leave it on for 30 minutes.
3. Rinse your hair thoroughly with Lemon Aid (see recipe on the previous page).

GINGER & TONIC

A nice pick-me-up, this potion will also add luster and shine to your curls. Vegetable glycerin can be found at most health food stores.

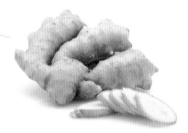

2 cups water
2 heaping tablespoons fresh grated ginger
1 teaspoon vegetable glycerin

1. Place the water in a medium pan, and heat over high until the water comes to a boil.
2. Add the ginger and the vegetable glycerin, bring the mixture back to a boil, and boil for 1 minute.
3. Cover the pot, turn off the heat, and let the ginger mixture steep until cool.
4. Strain the liquid to remove the ginger bits. Pour the Ginger & Tonic into bottles.
5. Pour liquid over wet hair as a prerinse before cleansing. Ginger & Tonic can also be used as a facial spritz or, if you leave out the vegetable glycerin, as a tea to aid digestion. (Just add lemon, lime, and agave or honey.)

The G & T potion can be refrigerated for up to 1 week.

Makes 2 cups Ginger & Tonic

GLISTEN TO ME

Spritz this gentle, all-natural hair spray on your curls whenever they look dull or need a quick pick-me-up. It will add shine and extra dimension. For this recipe, use distilled water because it doesn't contain minerals. Vegetable glycerin can be found at most health food stores.

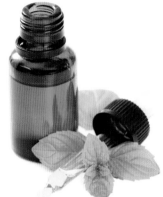

one 12-ounce spray bottle
12 ounces distilled water
3 drops favorite herbal essence
1 tablespoon vegetable glycerin

1. Fill the spray bottle with the distilled water.
2. Add the herbal essence and the vegetable glycerin to the water. Shake well.
3. This spritz is potent, so experiment with application and amount. You can spritz it over all of your hair or just apply it to individual strands of hair with your fingers.
4. Store the bottle in a cool place. It can last for up to 6 months.

WHATTA CURL WANTS

The baking soda in this recipe will remove heavy product buildup and leave your hair clean, shiny, and refreshed. It's a favorite of models and actresses.

1 tablespoon baking soda
1 cup hot water

1. Combine the baking soda and hot water, and stir to blend. Let the mixture cool.
2. Put the soda water in a spray bottle and shake.
3. Wet, condition, and blot-dry your hair as usual.
4. Spray or pour the soda water over your hair.
5. Leave it on your hair for 1 to 2 minutes, feel the sizzle, then rinse with cool water.
6. Cleanse your hair and/or condition, then style.

LOVE IS IN THE HAIR

This sensual mix of moisturizing oils acts as a refreshing tonic for dry, color-treated, thirsty curls. Jojoba oil, shea butter, and essential oils can be found at most health food stores.

4 tablespoons olive oil, jojoba oil, or shea butter
4 tablespoons conditioner
2 to 3 drops musk oil or other essential oil

1. Mix the olive oil, conditioner, and essential oil together well.
2. Apply the oil mixture to wet hair with your fingers, saturating all your curls.
3. Leave the oil on your hair overnight or for as long as you can.
4. Rinse hair thoroughly. Then cleanse and/or condition and style.

SUPER NATURAL NUTRIENT RINSE

This ancient remedy originally from Japan uses the nutrient-rich water that's left over after cooking pasta, rice, potatoes, quinoa, or soybeans to add extra shine and body without stripping the hair of its own oils.

cheesecloth or small burlap bag
1 to 2 handfuls of rice, pasta, potatoes, quinoa, or soybeans
2 quarts of water
1 tablespoon grated ginger or 1 drop of orange flower water

1. Fill cheesecloth, a burlap bag, or any perforated bag with uncooked rice, pasta, potatoes, quinoa, or soybeans, and tie the bag shut.
2. Place the bag in a pot, and add enough water to cover it.
3. Bring the water to a boil, and then let it simmer for 10 to 15 minutes.
4. Let the water cool, and then remove the bag from the pot. The infused water will feel slightly thicker than plain water.
5. Add ginger, orange flower water, or your choice of fragrance to the nutrient water.
6. Pour the nutrient water in bottles.
7. Use the nutrient water as a precleansing rinse by pouring it over your hair before cleansing, massaging it into the scalp, and then rinsing. Or pour it through your hair after rinsing out your sulfate-free cleanser, leave it on for a couple of minutes, and rinse your hair with regular water before applying a conditioner.
8. Store the nutrient water in the fridge for up to a week.

Makes nutrient water for a few treatments

curl confession

Patti Paige *owner of Baked Ideas*

When I was a little girl, I was so desperate for straight hair that moved when I turned my head that I begged my mother to buy me a bathing cap with a ponytail attached to it. For a while, my mother had my hair cut very short—I suppose to make it more manageable—and people thought I was a boy, which of course I hated. When it was longer, she'd tie it back in two tight pigtails, like a cartoon character.

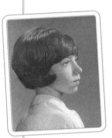

As a teenager, I tried everything to banish the curls. I'd slather Dippity-Do styling gel on my hair, then tape it down. I don't know where I got this idea, but somehow it made sense. When I'd remove the tape in the morning, I'd often strip away pieces of skin. Whenever I went to a hair salon, the stylist didn't have a clue. I would insist that she leave my hair long enough to "put it back in a ponytail," but I always left disappointed and upset.

Then I had my daughter, Dena. At age two she would cry in front of the mirror whenever she looked at her mop of dark ringlets. She'd also clip handkerchiefs to the sides of her head to pretend she had long, straight hair. I worried that she was learning this from me, so I decided then and there to wear my hair in curls—and not always tie it back. It took me until my late forties to accept my curls, but I'm happy to say that wasn't the case for Dena. She's now in her early twenties and likes her curls. The fact remains that my hair will always be something to contend with. But thanks to my daughter, I don't hide my ringlets.

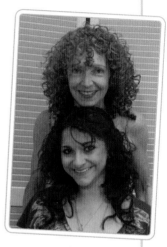

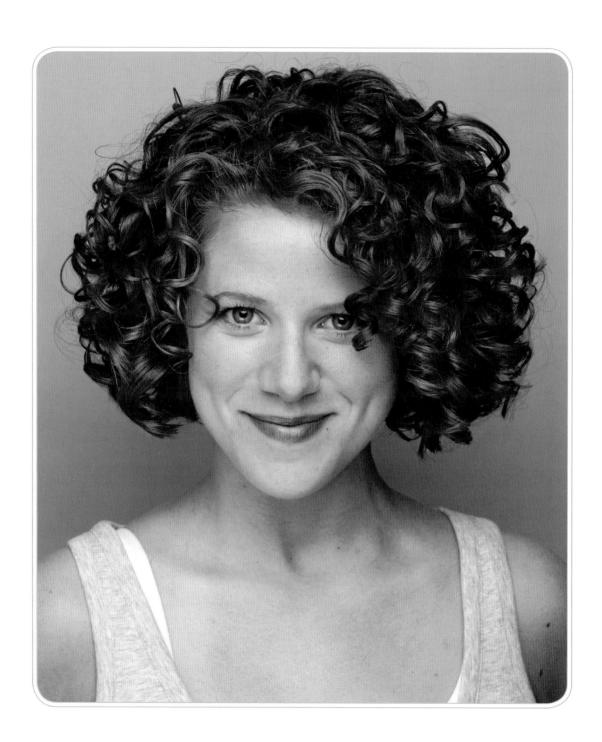

CHAPTER 9

a cutting-edge philosophy

Most curly girls have stories about abuse at the hands of hairstylists. We've asked for a trim and ended up completely shorn and looking like a skinned poodle. We've had stylists wet down our hair, then cut straight across as though it's straight, and the result is an unrecognizable spring-back of uneven, frizzy, angry curls. My clients have recounted tales of bad haircuts that were more traumatic than illnesses or surgeries they've had. Often, it's not only the constant bad cuts that scar the curly girl, but the emotional abuse, like having a stylist say, "What do you want me to do with *this*?"

A stylist must approach each head and each curl as a separate entity with a life of its own.

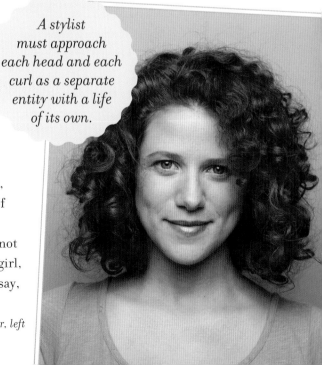

Before, and after, left

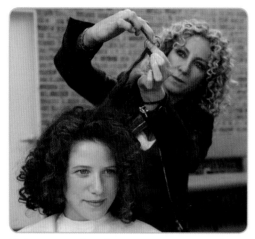

Make sure your hairdresser examines your curls.

I've gone home in tears after a haircut, so when a nervous client sits down in front of me for the first time, I can anticipate her fears. I understand her history so thoroughly, she might think I've been spying on her. (Whatever our backgrounds, curly girls share a universal past about our curls.) I begin by telling her that I'm going to give her a haircut that's just for her. Every curly person's hair is different—in the tightness of curls, how randomly the curls are distributed, and how they naturally frame the face. So you'll never find the right cut in one of those books of sample styles some salons pass around as if you're ordering from a Chinese menu. There is not a *style* for curly heads. I can't hand you a picture and say that's how you're going to look, unless it's a picture of you.

You've been blessed with hair that has a mind and life of its own. Every strand reacts differently to scissors. The stylist has to approach each curly girl individually, regarding her hair's texture, degrees of curliness, and how one curl relates to others around it. The most essential part of a curly haircut is to cut it when the hair is dry. In fact, cutting hair dry, whether it's naturally curly or naturally straight, makes lots of sense because that's how we wear our hair. And it's the *only* way to cut curly hair. Why?

Wet curls and dry curls are like Dr. Jekyll and Mr. Hyde. Moistened locks will actually fall into a different place than they will when they're dry. Curly hair may be halfway down your back when wet, only to spring up as much as 6 to 10 inches when it's dry. Imagine cutting fabric for a couture dress. You wouldn't wet the fabric and then cut it. It would expand when wet, and the dress would shrink when it dried. Hair is a fiber, too, as delicate as chiffon. Also, there are often several types of curls on one head and you can't see this variety when the hair is wet.

With each new client, I begin by examining her hair carefully. I pay attention to every movement, every contour, every characteristic. Is the hair frizzy? Dry? Stiff or crispy from too much gel or other product? Has it been

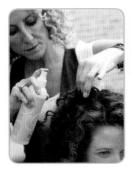 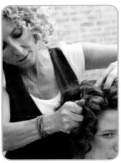

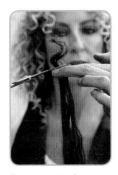

Trimming in the middle of a C curve.

straightened and dried out by blow-frying? Is the curl on the left side of the face tighter than the curl on the right side? I listen to the client, but I also allow the hair itself to guide me. I lightly spritz the hair with lavender spray and scrunch it gently so that I can figure out the client's type of curl. Sometimes, if the hair has been injured from years of blow-frying, it needs a thorough wetting, so I have the client's hair cleansed with conditioner, scrunched, and dried under a hood dryer or with a special curly hair diffuser. Only then do I begin the actual cutting.

Cutting curly hair is about what you leave, not what you snip off. Imagine each strand of hair lying in its rightful place as if it were a branch on a tree. I don't want to change it or manipulate it, just respond to it as it is. I look at each curl as a separate entity, noting any frayed ends.

What's your hair's natural length? It's that point when your curls flatter your face and fall gracefully. Some people need to grow out their curls to shoulder length before the natural pattern of their curl emerges. Others have curls that can be cut shorter. I ask the client what length she's happiest with and try to accommodate her preference. In general, it's better for the curly girl to leave her hair too long than too short. Any dramatic change requires a major consultation with the client first. We can always take more off, but we can't put it back on!

I decide on the amount that needs to be trimmed, then I cut at the beginning of each C of a curl to maintain its shape and

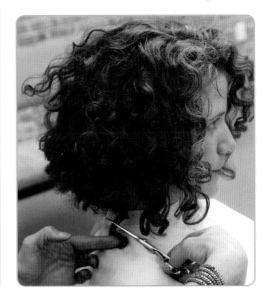

S's are consecutive C's reversed and sitting on top of each other. I cut at the beginning of each C.

avoid any dramatic spring-back. Think of a natural curl as an S shape. S's are consecutive C's reversed and sitting on top of each other. While I'm cutting, I stop and gently shake the curls from the root to see where they lie on top of each other and how they're going to fall when they're in motion—another factor you can't possibly see or predict when hair is wet.

After the initial haircut, most curly cuts are about mane-tenance. Basically, I

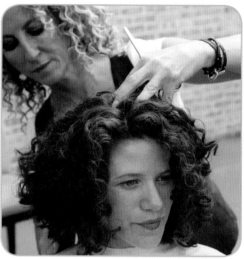

trim just the ends to oxygenize the hair, so they can take in and absorb more oxygen and water. If you are trying to grow your hair long or grow out relaxed hair, get frequent trims (see page 99).

curl your enthusiasm

Some of us are programmed to think it's time for a cut just because a specific period of time has passed. When that time comes, I suggest waiting a week before you make an appointment. Our curls can go through phases and act up for a few days, only to find their way again. If you want your hair to grow longer and have too frequent trims, you are in "yo-yo mode" because you are cutting your hair off before giving it a chance to grow. Instead, remember what your hair looked like six weeks before. Do you want to go forward or backward?

FINDING THE KINDEST CUTTER

One of the biggest complaints I hear from curly girls around the world is, "I can't find someone to cut my curls!" This doesn't surprise me. When it comes to curls, the beauty school curriculum is dated and archaic. The hair academy should have a whole wing dedicated to curl facts and the cutting and care of natural curls. But until that happens, here are some things to keep in mind before you let anyone approach your hair with a pair of scissors.

The surest way to find someone who cuts curly hair correctly is, of course, to see a haircutter's work. So when you spot someone with curly hair that looks wonderful, ask her where she has it cut. (Don't hesitate just because you think it's intrusive; most people will feel flattered.) If you live in a big city, you might flip through magazines for a style you like, then check the credits for the name of the salon or stylist. Otherwise, keep asking around until you find someone whose hair looks great.

Questions to Ask a Stylist

Before making an appointment, phone the salon and ask these questions:

☐ Is the stylist an expert at cutting curly hair?

☐ Does the stylist have naturally curly hair? Does she wear it curly? If so, this is a good sign; if the stylist's hair is blow-dried straight, ask for another stylist.

☐ Will the stylist see you before a cut for a consultation? Don't be offended if the answer is no; it could mean he's so popular that he has no time. Some places charge for a consultation.

☐ Does the salon offer the option of drying the hair under hooded dryers and diffusers rather than with blow-dryers? Explain that you want to keep your hair curly.

☐ Does the stylist cut curly hair while it's dry? If the answer is no, is she open to trying a different approach? Unless a stylist can see how much spring there is in your curls, she won't understand your hair and she's likely to cut too much when it's wet, only to discover that fact after your hair dries.

☐ What products does the salon use? If you don't use shampoo and have a favorite conditioner, bring it with you and politely ask them to use it. Most stylists won't object, especially if your hair is in good condition.

Let's assume you got all the right answers and have made an appointment. But if, when you arrive, you're told to change and get your hair shampooed, an alarm bell should go off in your head.

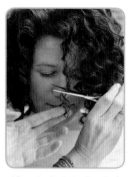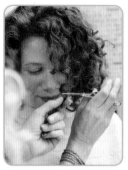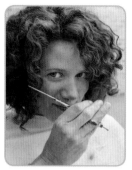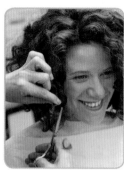

After the hair is dried, the stylist might handpick and cut a few curls around the face.

Instead, the stylist should sit you down, examine your hair, touch it, talk with you about your hair and what you envision having done—all before picking up the scissors. Pull a typical curl down to its farthest point and let go, so the stylist can see how tight the curl is. If your curls vary in tightness, show her which ones have a smaller spring factor. This is important so that she doesn't cut too much. Finally, explain that you'd rather leave your hair a bit too long than go too short.

Ideally, after the cut, the stylist should wet your hair and let it dry to see the finished results. This is the point when she makes those all-important final touches, picking up split ends that were missed the first time around or adjusting how the curls fall. You may want her to handpick and cut a few curls, especially around the front of your face. Don't be afraid to talk to the stylist about your preferences, as long as you're polite and diplomatic while being firm. After all, whose hair is it, anyway?

curl confession

Debbie Sable

My mother's generation liked the clean look of straight hair and even as a young child it was obvious that my mother didn't accept my curls. That had a huge effect on me. As an adult who finally learned to embrace her curls, I try to help several of the curly haired daughters of straight haired friends. I know how hard it is to have curly hair and that it's something that someone with straight hair can't understand. Recently, an eleven-year-old girl I'd helped thanked me profusely, and I felt such satisfaction. Her childhood with curly hair would be different than mine.

Pass This Along to Your Stylist

■ **DO** cut the hair when it is dry.

■ **DO** avoid blunt cuts, which ignore the spring factor and stretch the hair to an unnatural state so it's too short when it dries.

■ **DO** cut just before the crest of each curl or trim a few millimeters off the ends where they look frayed and knotty.

■ **DO** cut the top front of the hair last, and **DON'T** take too much off here because it's where the curls are shortest and most fragile.

■ **DON'T** thin out or debulk curly hair. The gravity and weight of the original curl formation is what gives hair its definition.

■ **DON'T** cut with a razor. Razors aren't as sharp as scissors, so they can create badly ripped and frayed ends.

■ **DON'T** brush, comb, or run fingers through curly hair when it's dry.

■ **DON'T** layer the hair too much unless you're cutting an advanced curly girl's hair.

Top Salon Crimes Committed Against Curly Girls

■ **Razoring, slicing, carving, thinning out, or debulking.** Razoring and thinning curls deforms the actual curl structure and makes the ends look ripped, frizzy, and weak. Since curly hair is almost weightless, this method reduces the hair to a bunch of fishhook strands—thicker at the carving point and very thin at the end of the slice. Plus it grows out terribly. Curls rely on a sharp scissor and a clean cut so the haircut lasts longer and the ends look healthy.

■ **Texturizing.** By "texturizing," salons mean they are going to slightly relax the hair without overstraightening it. But there's a very fine line here and it's very difficult to achieve. I don't recommend this

treatment, as it tends to leave the texture of the hair uneven and cause breakage—and oh, then there's the root grow-out in a couple of weeks, which just isn't pretty.

■ **Extensions.** These pieces of extra hair are sewn on to your existing hair. Extensions are pricey and time consuming and their weight can pull out your real hair and make your hairline recede so far back you look like Queen Elizabeth. (Extensions can also fall out at the most inopportune times. It's just not fun when someone says, "Excuse me, Miss. You dropped your hair," and, trust me, I've actually seen this happen—more than once!)

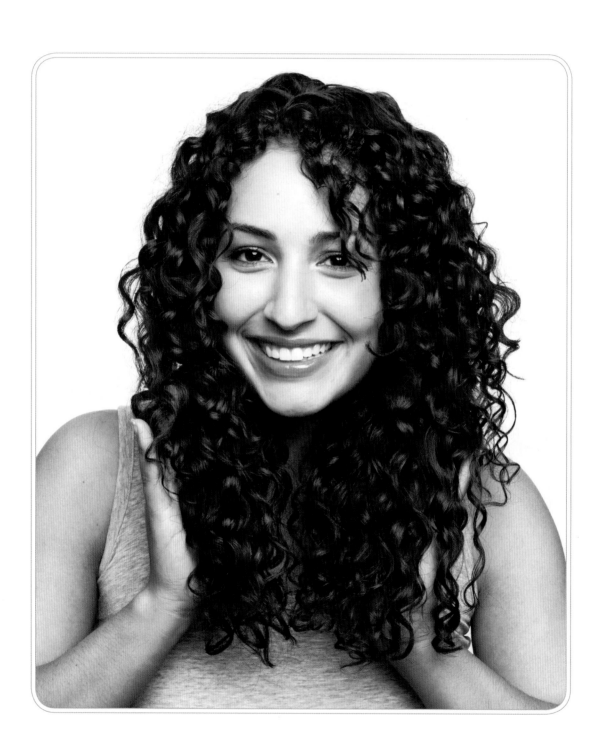

self-mane-tenance

TRIMMING YOUR OWN HAIR AFTER SHEAR FRUSTRATION

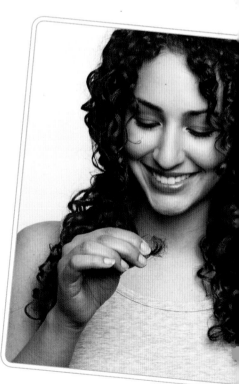

Suggesting that you cut your own hair—or someone else's—is a tricky subject if you're not a trained hairdresser. But throughout the years, many curly girls have asked me to teach self-mane-tenance and I understand why. After all, horrible haircuts are probably the most traumatic experiences in a curly girl's hair history. Myself included. At age sixteen, after going home in tears after yet another devastating haircut, I decided to take matters (and scissors) into my own hands. I felt like Scarlett O'Hara, when she shakes her fist and looks at the darkened sky, only I vowed, "As God is my witness, I will

When it comes to cutting curly hair, I always say, "It's not what you take off; it's what you leave on."

never let anyone else cut my hair again!" And I haven't since that day. If you're a curly girl, I know you can relate. We've all had the experience of sitting in the salon chair looking in the mirror, and with each snip, you see the haircut unfold as if you're witnessing a car wreck in slow motion. And, you're in it. Unfortunately, it can take months, even years, to recover from a cut where you end up completely shorn.

The sharpest point I want to make in this chapter is to teach you how to trim your own hair, or what I call "oxygenize" your curls yourself. You can do this in

THE TUNNEL CUT

Beware: There is a dreadful haircut that some stylists perform on thick, curly hair. It's sometimes called a "tunnel cut," but it has other aliases. They crop some curls at the roots and then leave a layer of longer hair over it, because they think this debulks the hair. But it actually makes the hair look bigger as the shorter pieces grow and push the longer, top layer outward. What a disaster! This was the last haircut I ever got many, many years ago. The aftermath looked like rats had gnarled on my hair!

between your regular haircuts, to save time and money or simply out of "shear" frustration at the haircuts that you've gotten. "Oxygenize" means to refresh and aerate, so that the ends of the hair strands can breathe in more oxygen and moisture. I'm not talking about cutting big chunks of hair or reshaping it—that's for your stylist. I'm talking about a fraction of an inch, half a C curl or, at most, a full C shape in your curl's spiral in order to remove the frayed, knotty, granular ends of your hair. (See page 94 for information on the C shapes of your curls.) With sharp, professional hair scissors, a small snip can go a long way for a curly do.

I think of trimming the hair the same way you'd trim trees or plants in the garden. Your eyes would go to the end of a stem or branch and instinctively cut off the part that looked gnarly and dried out. By pruning the plant or tree, you're helping it take in oxygen and water from the atmosphere. Almost immediately, it starts to look healthier and ready for new growth. Now, apply this same thinking to the ends of your hair, and you will be amazed at what a difference a little trim can and will make!

By now you know that curls are fragile and need to be cut with caution, and that cutting an inch off curly hair can look like you cut off three to four inches because of the spring factor. You may want to start with a professional cut from your favorite curly stylist, and then later just trim a tiny amount of hair where needed to maintain the style. When you are at the salon, watch how your stylist cuts your hair when it is dry, and pick up some tips.

Before doing anything, it's important to buy a pair of quality scissors that are made specifically for cutting hair. These usually cost upward of $100 at a beauty supply store or online. This may sound pricey, but believe me, it's worth the investment. What you don't want to use is a pair of thinning shears or a razor that will fray and split the ends of the hair. (If you have a trusted stylist, you can ask her what type of scissors she uses. My all-time favorite brand is Hikari.)

You also need a mirror, good lighting, and a neutral background so you can see the silhouette and shape of your hair. Lastly, you'll need a hand mirror that's big enough to help you see the back of your hair. Make sure that your hair has been cleansed and styled according to the Curly Girl Method for your curl type. This doesn't have to happen immediately before you trim your hair. I like to cleanse my curls in the morning and then trim them before bed, because by then my hair is totally dry and my curls fall naturally.

A word of caution: Never cut your

scissors

The right scissors are key to a great curly cut. If a superior cutting tool is used, the scissors melt through the hair in silence with precision and accuracy, and the haircut will grow out with no split ends. Scissors made for fabric or paper won't give hair a precise cut. In fact, these and other inferior scissors can actually fray the ends because they tend to be duller than hairdressing scissors. Dull scissors will make a gnawing or grinding sound when you cut, and can require that you cut your curls a couple of times to get through the hair because they latch and pull.

Once you get a good pair of hair scissors, don't use them for anything other than hair. Carefully wipe the scissors with a bit of olive oil and a chamois cloth after use. Store them safely between trims. (They're very sharp, so don't leave them around for children or pets to find.) A quality pair of shears will last a lifetime, and will stay sharp since they're being used only on your hair (unlike those at a salon where they are used on thousands of heads of hair).

Quality hairdressing scissors are worth the investment.

hair when it is wet. Never cut it while you're in the dark, in a moving vehicle (trust me, people do this), or drinking alcohol. Also make sure you have plenty of time to cut your hair; when you're rushed you're more likely to make mistakes. And be careful: high-quality hairdressing shears are very sharp, so it's easy to snip your fingers along with your hair.

CURLY GIRL

GUIDE FOR SELF-MANE-TENANCE

First, stand in front of a mirror and look carefully at your hair's overall shape and the ends of the hair, which you're going to trim. Then, take a handheld mirror and turn so the back of your head is toward the wall mirror and you're holding the hand mirror in front of you. Look at the way the hair looks and falls in the back of your head and look again at the ends that you're going to trim.

Even though you are trimming only the very

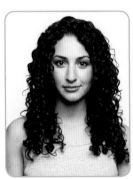

ends of the hair, it's important that your scissors feel comfortable in your hands. A couple of cautions: Don't open the blades too wide so the scissors look like a big X, because this may result in taking off bigger chunks of hair than desired. And don't hold the scissors facing downward like a plane plunging nose first to the ground, as this will shred and fray the hair. Make a clean cut across the dry hair.

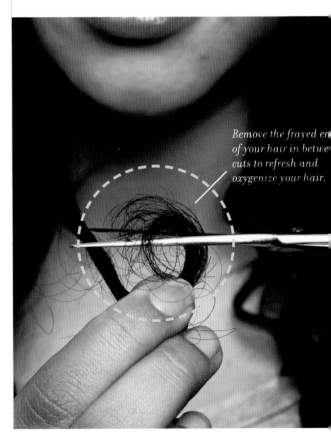

Remove the frayed en of your hair in betwe cuts to refresh and oxygenize your hair.

Trimming the Sides

TO START... shake your curls by swaying your head back and forth. This allows them to naturally position themselves.

1 If your hair is shoulder length or longer, part the hair in the back and bring both sides forward in front of your shoulders as though you were going to make pigtails.

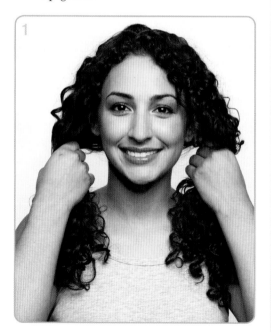

2 Look carefully at the ends to decide where you plan to trim.

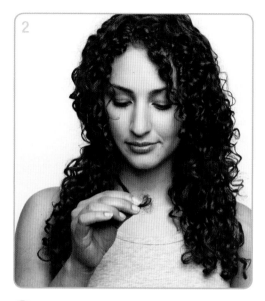

3 Take your first defined curl unit, and hold it between your thumb and your index and middle fingers so that the bottom of your fingers targets where you want to cut.

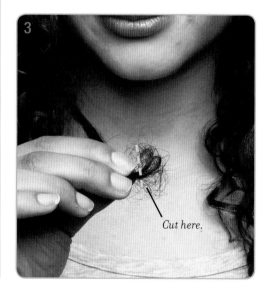

Cut here.

4 Then, hold the scissors in your other hand, and snip the end of the curl unit with the tip of the blades. Cut straight across. This kind of trimming will get rid of frayed, knotted ends.

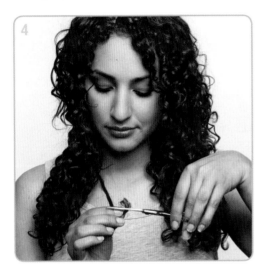

5 Continue to do the same on each curl unit on that side of your head, trimming off about equal amounts of hair on each one. Avoid combing or running your fingers through your hair, which would disrupt your curl's intrinsic shape.

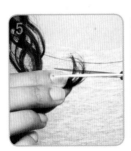 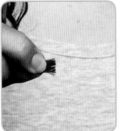

Cut hair straight across.

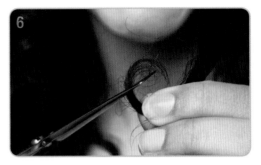

6 Next, trim the hair on the other side of the head in the same manner.

7 Shake your curls, and then examine your newly trimmed hair. Note any uneven locks, and give those a snip in the same way.

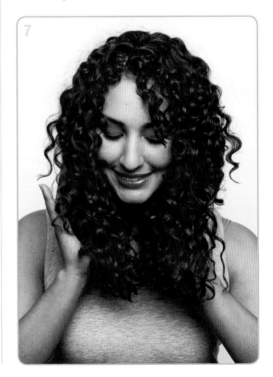

curl confession

Netta Rabin *children's book designer*

More times than I can count, my long curls were cut to an awkward shoulder length because the hairdresser cut my hair wet, making it shrink up when it dried. My first good haircut was at a curly hair salon, and it was a life-changing experience! For the first time, I felt blessed to have curly hair. I finally embraced having hair that changes every day and has a life of its own. I realized that my hair was an extension of my personality.

After being a dedicated curly girl for ten years, I started cutting my own hair, partly to save money and partly because my wedding was coming up and I was worried that even a professional curly stylist would cut my hair too short or mess up my bangs. My first self-trim looked pretty good. (The one thing I didn't realize was how important it is to use high-quality shears. I made the mistake of using household scissors, which frayed my hair a bit.)

Then, I cut my own bangs. I'd always wished I could have bangs, but thought curly ones looked ridiculous. That was until I saw the most adorable curly-banged waitress in my neighborhood restaurant. There was no way I was going to wait for an appointment at the salon; I wanted bangs right away. That night, I started cutting, and it was so much fun that I kept going until I had the big, crazy hair I was always afraid to ask my hairdresser to do. It's empowering to know I can trim my own hair to keep it healthy, and it's also saved me a lot of money.

And I loved how my hair turned out on my wedding day. Kudos to my stylist—myself.

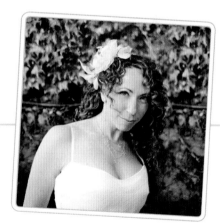

Trimming the Canopy

TOP LAYER OF HAIR ALL AROUND THE HEAD

1 Look in the mirror and imagine an invisible clock behind your head.

Raise hair upward so it's in line with the 12 o'clock position on your imaginary clock.

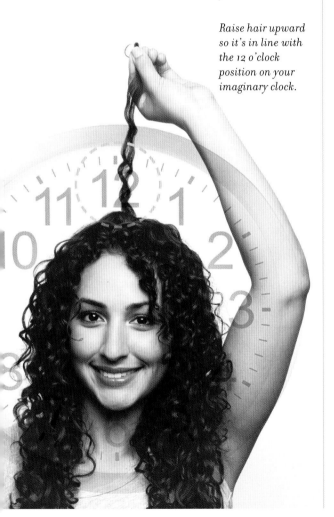

2 Starting with a curl from the canopy that's on the top of the crown, take the hair from the end of a curl unit and gently hold it between your thumb and your index and middle fingers.

3 Without putting any tension on the curl unit, raise it upward so it's in line with the 12 o'clock position on your imaginary clock. Hold it up as far as its length allows, perpendicular to the scalp, without pulling on it, and place it between your index and middle fingers at the point where you plan to trim the ends. Pull hair forward.

4 Carefully snip off the end of the hair that is anchored between your fingers with the tip of the scissors.

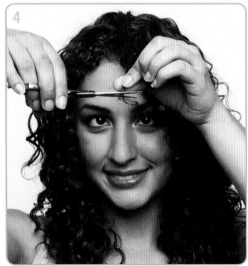

5 Next, do the same on the neighboring curl unit—which would be at 1 o'clock on your imaginary clock—on the left side of your head, and snip the end of that. Continue with the rest of the curl units on the left side of your head (which would be at 2 and 3 o'clock).

6 Now go back to the center of the back of the head, and trim the curls on the canopy of the hair on the right side of the head (which would be at 11, 10, and 9 o'clock).

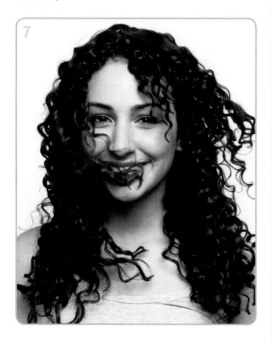

7 Occasionally, sway your hair back and forth to see how the trim looks in motion.

Trimming Hair in the Back

BENEATH THE CANOPY

1 Face away from the wall mirror, and, using the handheld mirror, position yourself so you see the back of your hair.

2 Sway your head back and forth to see how the back of your hair lies in relation to the sides. You may see a V shape where the sides are shorter than the hair in the back. If you like it, great. But if you want to trim the bottom end of the V to match the sides, you'll need to trim off a little more hair than just the very ends.

3 With your index and middle fingers, pick up the chosen curl unit from the center of the back beneath the canopy, and bring it around to the front on your right shoulder.

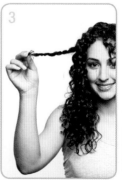 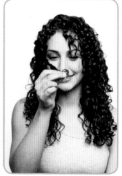

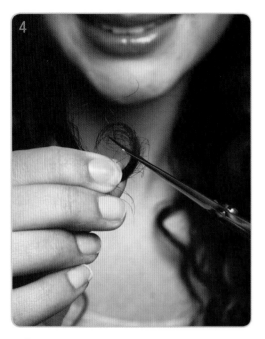

naturally. This way you'll see what other curls need trimming.

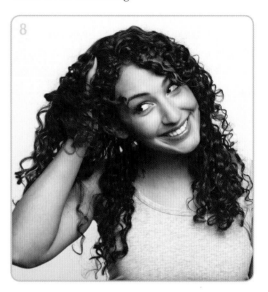

4 Position your fingers right above the area you want to trim. Avoid applying too much tension on the chosen curl unit, so you don't distort its actual length and therefore snip too much.

5 Cut the hair straight across at that point right above your fingers.

6 Take the curl unit next to it and repeat the above steps. Alternate doing the same thing from the center back on the right side.

7 Occasionally during the trim, shake your curls at the roots with your fingers so the newly cut hair falls

Trimming the Bangs

Bangs seem to grow out faster than hair on the rest of the head, so it's often the place you want to trim between cuts. Just be careful when trimming this area, since cutting too much can leave you with bangs that are too short, a style that doesn't usually work on curly hair unless you want a funky look. (As you well know, curly hair is quite moody, so some days the curls on your forehead contract while other days your bangs appear longer, which do not look as good framing your face.)

Make sure you hold the scissors gently and with ease and apply no tension to the hair. With bangs, err on the side of trimming less rather than more. I know I've said it before, but you can't add hair back if you cut it too short. Also, if you have a very prominent part or cowlick, keep in mind where it is.

1 Stand very close to the mirror. Unlike the rest of your hair, where you hold each curl with one hand while you trim with the other, you're going to trim your bangs without holding the hair. With this free-hand approach, your hair is lying in its natural position, and you can gauge exactly where to trim it.

2 Starting with the bang section that is in the middle of your forehead, pinch the curl unit from the root and lift it up slightly to see what it would look like when you cut it. Then place the scissors at the spot where you plan to trim.

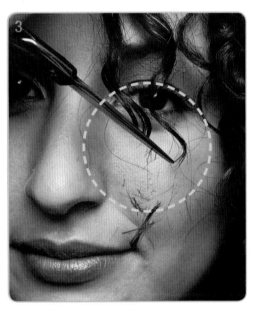

Snip the hair at the end of the curl unit or slightly below the beginning of the C curve.

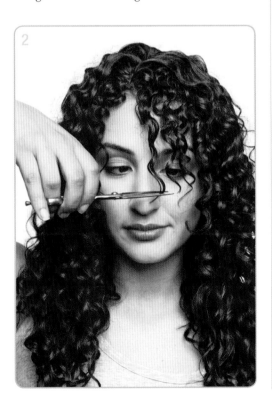

3 Hold the scissors gently and with ease. Carefully snip the hair at the end of the bang unit or slightly below the beginning of the C curve.

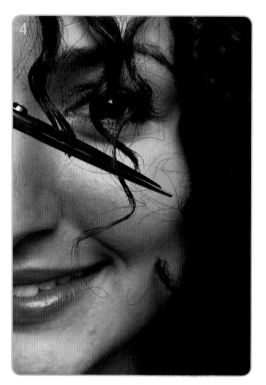

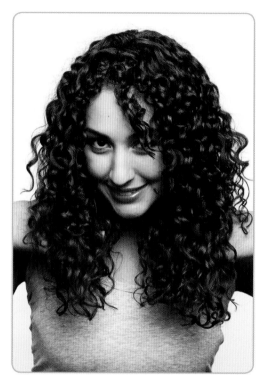

4 Move on to the curl unit lying next to the curl in the middle of the forehead. Trim it at the beginning of the C, leaving it slightly longer than the strand you just cut.

5 Continue cutting the neighboring strands as though you are going down a staircase. If you have bangs on both sides, cut in this same way on the other side of the first bang section that you cut in the middle of your forehead.

When you've finished trimming your hair, check that the cut feels and looks visually connected. Take sections of hair from opposite sides of your head and gently bring them forward between your fingers toward the front of your face so you can see that the lengths are about even and that all the ends have been freshly trimmed. Ends you missed will look obvious as the newly trimmed hair exposes the frayed strands like a neon light. Also, note that as your hair settles in the next few days, you may see a couple of pieces that need a snip.

curl confession

Denise McCoy *stay-at-home mother*

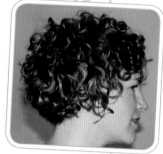

I could never figure out what to do with the kinky curly hair I got once I hit puberty. I can't count how many hairstylists said that their way of cutting it would be the solution. It never was. Most of the time it just made my hair worse.

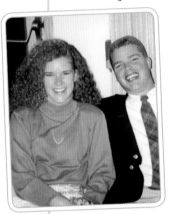

Then a few years ago a friend called me from Dallas. "This is a bit awkward," she warned. "But there's a girl in my office whose hair is so unruly we make fun of it. Then she came in today and her hair was jaw-dropping gorgeous. I thought of you." I didn't even think to be insulted; I wanted to know this girl's secret, which was the book *Curly Girl.* I started to follow the routine and I began to love my hair.

But I needed to find someone to cut my curls. I met Lorraine on a trip to New York, and when I told her that I lived in Texas and had trouble finding someone I could trust with my curls, she taught me to cut them myself. I've been doing this for four years. Occasionally, I'll have my colorist trim my hair in the back, but the whole time I'm directing her exactly where to cut. It took me a while to get the courage up to tell her she couldn't cut my hair wet. But she didn't think that was a big deal. Now, I not only cut my own hair, but I set up shop on my back porch and cut a few friends' curls, too!

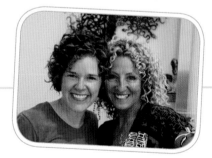

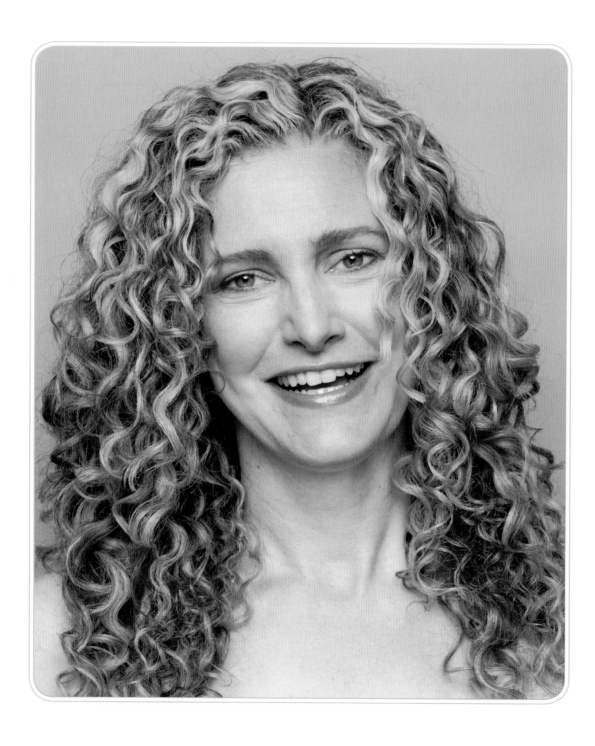

CHAPTER 11

color
me curly

IT'S ALL ABOUT HUE!

C ontrary to what many people believe, color and curls *do* mix, especially with today's available color processes that can keep hair healthy looking. You just have to take into account the special needs of curly hair and use color sensibly. Curly hair absorbs damaging chemicals more easily because the cuticle around the hair shaft is open. "It also takes longer to recover from any damage, because curly hair is so porous," says Denis DaSilva, co-owner of Devachan.

Denis and the DevaColor team agree that semipermanent and demipermanent colors are the best choices for curly hair, actually for all hair. Semipermanent color is not as damaging to the hair because it doesn't remove any of the natural color. Demipermanent color is more effective on gray hair, which may resist a milder coloring

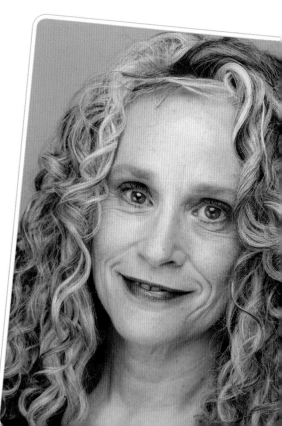

process. "The best time to use permanent color, which offers more coverage, is on very hydrated, healthy hair," says Larry Bianco, a DevaColor expert. "But if hair is dehydrated, any chemical process will deteriorate the hair fiber even more. Not only will the hair be unhealthy, your color won't look good." The fewer ammonia-based products you use on your hair, the less dehydrated it becomes.

At Devachan, we usually recommend that clients come back every four to six weeks for color. But that time frame depends on how fast your hair grows, your personal tolerance for exposed roots, and how close your artificial color is to your natural shade. Roots that are close in shade to your colored hair won't be as noticeable, while those that are drastically different in color will create an obvious line of demarcation like a landing strip (see page 147 for a hair pinning technique to help hide roots).

When it comes to choosing a color, we advise clients to avoid dramatic color transformations overnight. Start with a demi- or semipermanent color that's close to your own or two or three tones lighter. Live with that color for a while before doing anything more drastic. Remember that the depth and dimension of color will change as the curls return to their natural state. As I often tell my

clients, blond shouldn't be built in a day. If you want to go from dark brown to blond, build in the color gradually. I began by having a few handpicked curls highlighted. I loved the results and the positive feedback I was getting, so I gradually added more . . . naturally!

Curly girls can also have fun playing with highlights a few shades brighter than their natural color. At Devachan, we specialize in Pintura, a highlighting technique that Denis invented. "Here, the colorist picks out the more raised three-dimensional pieces of hair, which best reflect light, and paints highlights onto dry hair curl by curl," Denis says. "This brings attention to certain parts of the curl and creates dimension, something curly hair needs, by putting light in an area where there naturally is none."

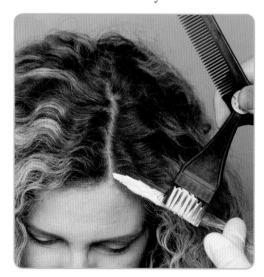

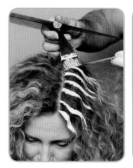 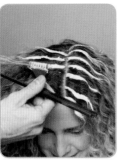

The Pintura technique also gives the colorist more control over where he or she places the highlights. By painting them on deliberately and individually, you're guaranteed perfect placement from roots to the ends and you'll see the highlights exactly where they've been applied.

"This control is important because placement matters when it comes to curly hair," says Edward Fagley, a DevaColor expert. If highlights are too close together and they overlap on previously colored hair, which happens if the traditional foil method of highlighting is used, then you lose dimension. But with the Pintura method, you can leave just enough space between each curl to create a ribbon of light and dimension. Highlighting using foil can also bake and break curly hair, which is fragile.

If you're an advanced curly girl, then you have what I call a healthy foundation of hydration. You don't have to do anything different before getting your

hair colored because your hair is already conditioned. But if you haven't been doing the Curly Girl Method yet, start to condition your hair daily a few weeks before getting color. It's like priming a wall before painting so you get better results. Also, steer clear of detergent-filled shampoos. If you're opting for a new style, or getting your hair trimmed or shaped, have your hair cut first and while it's dry, because the shape of the cut helps determine the color placement.

"Only two people should know that I color my hair. My haircolorist and me."
—CORNELIA PECKMAN

SKIP THE GLOSSES

Many salons offer treatments called glosses and glazes that promise you a head full of shiny hair. "But in my opinion," Larry says, "gloss is something that goes on a car and glaze goes on a doughnut." In general, curly hair just isn't as shiny as straight hair. Straight hair lies flat, so light can bounce off its smooth surface, making it shine. But curly hair's more porous surface and concave areas don't reflect as much light. Glosses and glazes can also clog the hair's cuticle, making it difficult to hydrate the hair properly afterward. The best way to get your hair looking its shiniest is to follow the Curly Girl Method so that hair is well hydrated.

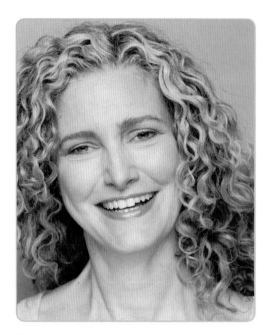

SILVER SIRENS

A lot of clients ask how they can keep their gray hair but make it look beautiful. The first thing I tell them is that silver foxy hair *is* beautiful. It can be elegant and it is sexy. The problem seems to be with the word *gray*, which has a social stigma implying old or worn, especially when it comes to women. My first piece of advice is to change the way you think about your strands. Call them "silver" and think of them as natural and beautiful.

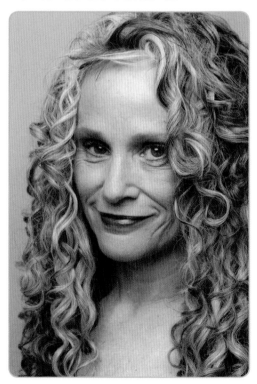

Then do your part, by coming to the salon with your curls as you usually wear them, so the stylist and colorist can see your hair in its most natural state.

After you get color, treat your hair with special TLC (Tender Loving Conditioning), using one of the moisturizing treatments recommended in chapter 8 (see page 77). All hair, but particularly curly hair, takes a few days to settle after being color-treated. The depth perception and dimension of color will blend and look amazing in no time, especially when you're a shampoo-free curly girl. Remember that the more often you shampoo your hair, the more quickly the color will fade.

curl confession

Sandra Gering *art dealer*

At the age of sixty-one, when I was diagnosed with breast cancer, I shaved off all my hair rather than enduring the pain of watching it fall out from chemotherapy. As soon as I was done with chemo, the hair I'd lost started to grow back. Except now, instead of wavy platinum-blond hair, it was baby curls that were silver.

I didn't know how to handle my new hair, so I looked to my curly haired friends for direction. After using the right products, my hair came back strong, shiny, and thick, and it looked so good that I decided to leave it natural. I constantly get compliments on how pretty the silver color is. When one old friend suggested I go back to being a blonde, I told him I was no longer that person. I am who I am now and I like the naturalness.

Soon after my hair grew back, I went to Italy on vacation. There I met a much younger man—he was thirty-seven years old—who became my lover. I think my curls helped attract him. It was wonderful, and our romance lasted for two years.

"When I tell clients that their gray hair is beautiful, I instantly see a shift in their outlook," Larry says. And the best way to make your silver hair look better is to give it a foundation of hydration. "In reality, it's not the color of the hair fiber that makes it beautiful, it's the *quality* of the fiber. If hair is dehydrated, the tone and color change. So if you've been taking care of your hair by doing all the things we talk about in this book, automatically your silver hair will look better."

"If you want to go natural," Larry says, "focus on caring for your hair so that you can wean yourself off of color." The other thing that affects how good your silver strands look is your hairstyle (or lack thereof). For example, if you have long, gray, straggly strands, your hair will have a dated appearance. But if your very hydrated silver hair has a stylish cut, it'll look fabulous and, yes, youthful!

THE NATURAL HUE:

INTER-GRAY-TION

Another question clients often ask is how they can make the transition from colored hair to their natural hue. "Coloring can be an addiction, so you may have to wean off of it gradually," Larry explains. "You can do this by coloring less in one way or another." To do that:

■ Stop using permanent color. Instead, opt for demi- or semipermanent color, which doesn't cover hair as fully so you will begin to see a gradual hint of your natural hair color. As a result, when roots come in there will be less of a line of demarcation than there is with permanent color, so your natural hue will be less shocking.

■ Another way to get used to going natural is to color most of your hair but leave some uncolored. A piece of hair in the front is a good place to try this, because you're faced with your natural hue daily and begin to get used to it.

■ Rather than having hair colored completely, you can have it colored with highlights, using the Pintura technique (see page 114). Painting color on your natural hair will cover some of it but not all. For a dramatic effect, you can "add some pepper to the salt," says Larry, by painting pieces of hair darker and leaving the rest white or silver.

■ Or you can go lighter in terms of the hue you color with. Going lighter better mimics what nature is doing as you age. Coloring with a lighter hue is an especially good idea if 75 percent or more of your hair is silver or white, because as hair grows in, there's not a big contrast between your roots and your colored hair. And because your skin tone also changes as your hair gets gray, your complexion will be more compatible with a lighter hair shade.

TOO YOUNG TO DYE

When clients ask colorist Michael Flores what to say to their tween or teen daughters who want highlights, he sees the daughter for a consultation. Then he explains that highlights require touch-ups every four to six weeks, that they can cause dryness, and that they are pricey. "I insist that the child pays for her hair coloring," says Michael. "She needs to know this is something you don't get free for the rest of your life and that it's a responsibility. Then if she still wants it, I make her wait until she's fifteen."

curly color care iss-hues

Michael Flores, owner of the Michael Flores Salon in Dallas, Texas, is concerned that a lot of colorists treat curly hair the same way as straight hair, which you simply can't do. Here are Michael's top tips:

■ **Beware of the brush.** If your colorist picks up a brush or comb when you sit in their chair, they're going to treat your curls like straight hair. That's a big mistake, and you should get up and walk out.

■ **Don't go straight.** Never let a colorist blow out your hair to color it. If they do, they'll be placing the color in areas that work for straight strands, not curly. Likewise, don't let your colorist blow your hair straight after getting it colored. Some say this helps them see the color they've just applied to your hair. But this makes no sense if your hair was colored for you to wear curly. Plus, the damaging heat is a third strike against your hair after it's been assaulted with color and shampoo.

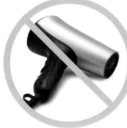

■ **Ask for the minimum.** The ammonia and peroxide in hair color and bleach can be very dehydrating to already dry, curly hair, so don't be afraid to tell your colorist that you want the minimum amount of ammonia and peroxide used. (They do need to use some.)

■ **Get real.** Have realistic expectations about the kinds of color your curly strands can take. For example, you can't be a double-processed blond and have healthy, pretty, curly hair. These two processes use high amounts of bleach and ammonia, so rather than being bouncy and shiny, your hair will probably look like yellow hay. (That is, if it doesn't break off from all those drying chemicals!)

■ **Just touch-up.** If you have only a few gray strands, apply color only to them.

■ **Say no to the poo.** Shampooing hair after a color application removes some of the color that was just applied and ruffles the cuticle so the hair looks dull and dry.

If you get your hair colored at the salon, protect all the good work and money you're spending by bringing your own no-poo. Just take a bottle with no label on it and fill it with a sulfate-free cleanser or conditioner. Tell your colorist that you have a sensitive scalp and that your doctor says you must use this after coloring. After all, if you don't protect your hair, who will?

DIY OR DYE

Ten Things to Do Before You DYE

Coloring your own hair isn't as easy as it looks on TV commercials. You really need an artistic hand and a discerning eye. Plus, many of the at-home coloring kits have high concentrations of chemicals, which put your already dry curls at risk. Make a mistake and it takes longer for curly hair to recover from lost moisture. That said, an estimated 65 percent of women who color their hair do so at home, so I want to offer you some tips for doing it safely:

■ Avoid permanent color. Use only semipermanent or demipermanent color. With these, you're less likely to make a mistake, or if you do, it will eventually wash out. Plus, semi- and demipermanent color cover gray hair well, give a gentle lift to your natural color, and enhance shine without damaging hair.

■ Avoid "sun-activated" highlights. They'll turn your hair orange!

■ Don't go more than two shades darker or one shade lighter than your existing color. Go for a neutral shade because you're less likely to have a mishap. If you want a major color change, have it done by a professional colorist.

■ If you highlight at home, have a friend help you. (And save the cocktails for later.) Look for a highlighting kit that contains a wand or brush that makes it easy to paint highlights on individual curls.

■ When doing your roots, make sure not to overlap the new color onto the old color. "Apply color just to the roots or you'll get a dark band in the overlap area," says colorist Edward Fagley.

■ Don't run color all the way down to the ends. Some people say this refreshes them, but all it does is darken them.

■ Leave on hair color for less time than what's recommended on the box and never leave it on longer. Your hair will grab enough color, but you won't have those damaging chemicals on your hair as long.

■ If your curls look straighter after coloring, that's not a good sign. It means the hair has been overprocessed and may have overlapped color.

■ To see a truer color, go outdoors to look at it. Natural light will give you a better read of what your hair looks like than indoor fluorescent lighting.

■ Know that semipermanent, demipermanent, and permanent color will not lift a previous color application. For instance, if your hair has been colored a light brown, you can't make it lighter by adding an even lighter shade of brown. Only a professional colorist can make your hair lighter by using a professional color-removing process.

curl confession

Nathalie Wechsler *freelance illustrator, painter, and owner of a paper products company*

When I was growing up, I was obsessed with the story of Rapunzel and her long hair. I loved giving my long-haired dolls different hairstyles, because my parents forced me to keep my own hair short. They thought curls were meant to be tamed. There is something about lots of curly hair that's very sexual, and parents don't like to see that in their kids. My parents wanted me to behave like a nice, quiet girl from a good family. So I kept my hair "quiet," but I rebelled in other ways.

Then as soon as I was out on my own, I let my hair grow out and go wild. I now think that my fascination with Rapunzel's hair had to do with becoming powerful and feeling in control. Rapunzel's long hair gave her the power to escape from the tower. I grew my hair long when my parents were no longer able to control me—or my curls.

Today, people are fascinated by my curls; strangers stop me on the street, and many even ask if they can touch the curls. Finally, now that I'm in my forties, my parents accept my hair. But that was pretty recent. Just a few years ago, I'd be talking to my father, and he'd stop me and say, "Get your hair out of your face."

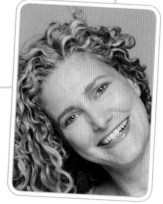

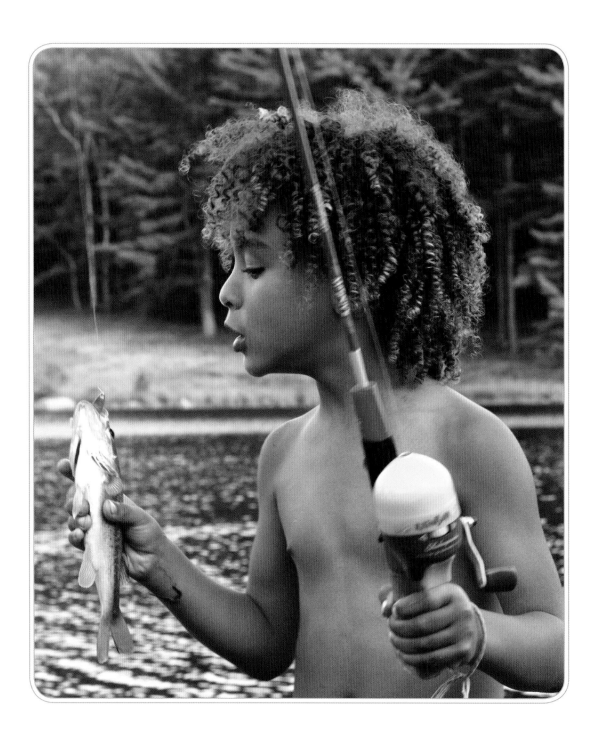

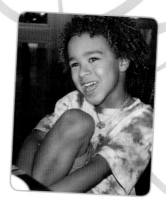

CHAPTER 12

curly kids

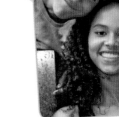

caring for underage curls

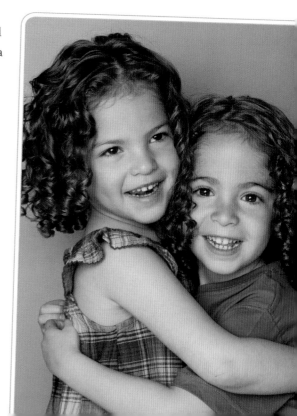

Children don't come with instructions and neither does their hair. But if you've got a curly kid, knowing how to care for his or her hair can make life for you and your child a lot easier. My clients frequently tell me that they hated their curls from a very young age and that much of their childhood angst stemmed from their strands. Many curly girls and boys recount the physical *and* emotional pain of having mothers who didn't know how to handle their curls. They would straighten, braid, or brush their child's hair, trying to untangle what they saw as knots, or in total frustration, they'd cut it off completely. Early in life, these curly kids got the message that their hair was not acceptable—that it was something to control and hide, not embrace and love.

Thankfully, the curly life doesn't have to be that way for curly kids anymore. Just as we want our children to grow up feeling good about themselves, we also want them to grow up feeling good about their hair. Those swirling strands affect our children's self-esteem on a daily basis. Honor and care for your child's curls and you will teach him or her to do the same.

Of course, if you're the parent of curly haired kids, as I am, or if you've been one yourself, you know that underage curls can get into more messes than a two year old with a bucket of goo. Kids are constantly running, tumbling, swinging, and jumping into mud puddles and piles of leaves. They throw sand at each other. They have food fights. They put on dress-up costumes, winter caps, bathing caps, and baseball hats, and never worry about whether their curls get matted or snarled. That is until it comes time to wash those curls, and then oceans of tears get washed down the drain along with the sand and dirt.

I recommend treating kids' curly hair the same way I treat adults' hair: with no shampoo, no brushes, and loads of conditioner. Surprisingly, even baby shampoos can contain harsh detergents, ingredients that aren't good for your child's delicate hair and scalp. And shampoos that promise to be "tear-free" can make you weep, since any foreign matter can make your eyes water. Plus, all that lathering up doesn't clean but ruffles the hair cuticle, which leads to more snarls. Instead, look for a sulfate-free cleanser or, if you can't find one, a botanical conditioner to cleanse with. (See page 77 for information on finding the right products.) Then, follow the steps below to cleanse your child's hair. Explain what you're doing, so kids'll know what to do when they start taking care of their own hair.

1 Have your child sit in the tub and tell him or her to look up at the ceiling. Use a plastic jug to gently and evenly pour water through the hair, wetting it thoroughly.

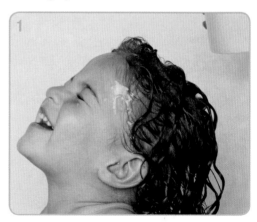

2 Cup one hand and apply a sulfate-free cleanser or botanical conditioner along the pads of your fingers. (If your

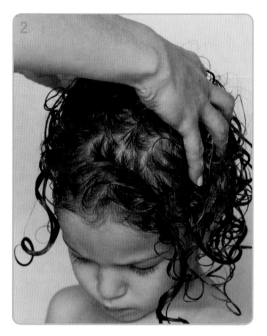

thoroughly. If possible, cup the hair in your hands, allowing the water to flow through them like a sieve, which helps protect the curl formation.

4 Put a shallow palmful of botanical conditioner in your hand, rub your hands together, and evenly smooth the conditioner on the canopy of your child's hair as though you are icing a cake. (The amount will vary. Older girls with long, thick curls will need more conditioner than a younger child with short, fine hair.) Gently use your fingers to work the conditioner through the wet hair, beginning at the ends and making your way up to separate tangles.

child has baby-fine hair, perhaps as little as ¼ teaspoon.) Evenly distribute the cleanser to the fingertips of your other hand. Then use firm, circular motions of your fingertips to massage your child's scalp. The cleanser combined with the stimulation from your fingers will emulsify and break down dirt particles and deodorize the scalp. It will also soften the hair and leave it knot free.

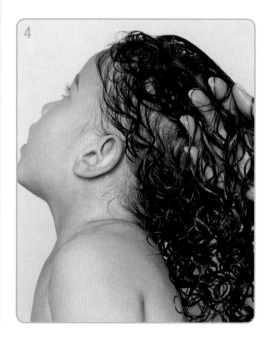

3 Again, ask your child to look up at the ceiling, and use a jug to pour water through the hair to rinse it

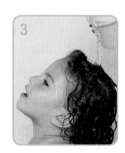

5 Apply an additional dollop of conditioner, about the size of a nickel, under the hair at the nape of the neck, the spot most prone to tangles and knots. That hair breaks easily, so be gentle when trying to release any tangles or knots. The hair should now feel smooth and silky—almost like wet seaweed.

6 Rinse the hair lightly so you leave some conditioner behind. You can do this by cupping your hands under the bath's running water and just splashing water over the canopy of the hair. Then use your hands to lightly squeeze the hair upward toward the roots to remove excess conditioner. (If your child's hair has a high frizz factor, don't rinse after conditioning.)

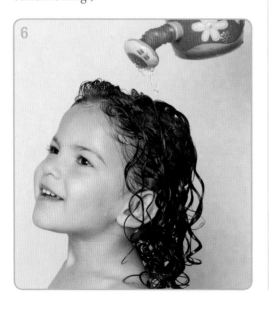

7 Once your little one is out of the bath, ask her to tilt her head upside down. Cup the hair with a microfiber towel, paper towel, or old cotton T-shirt, and scrunch-squeeze the hair upward toward the roots. This removes a little bit more conditioner but allows the hair to retain what it needs.

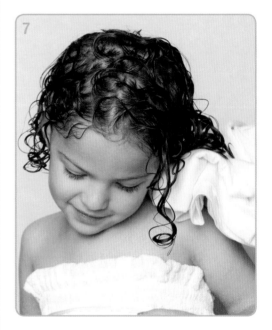

8 Gel isn't a must for kids' hair. Their hair is naturally healthier and more hydrated than adults' hair. But if your child has a high frizz factor, or for special occasions, you can apply a small amount of gel that is free of silicone, alcohol, and parabens to the canopy of the hair in a downward motion.

STICKY SITUATIONS

What happens when your curly kid gets glue, paste, food, or a wad of gum in his hair? Rub the area with an ice cube until the stickiness hardens and begins to crumble. Then make a paste out of a few drops of vinegar and about ¼ teaspoon of conditioner, and apply it to the matted spot. Let it soak in. Gently work the mess out with your fingers or with the end of a knitting needle.

Kids' curls don't need a daily cleansing. Lavender spray is great in the morning when your kids wake up with ruffled hair and you don't want to cleanse or fully wet their hair. Or you can just spritz their hair with a detangling spray made by combining equal amounts of water and conditioner in a spray bottle. I also use lavender spray to deodorize and reorganize my kids' curls after a day at the beach. (A little-known side benefit for school-age kids is that lavender is a good deterrent against lice.)

If your curly haired daughter insists on wearing her hair straight, comb it with your fingers and put it in a ponytail to dry. Or braid the hair while it's still wet, which will help eliminate frizz, but do not pull too tightly.

When it comes to cutting your child's curly hair, it's best to follow its intrinsic shape, whether it's waves, ringlets, or smaller curls, and let your child wear a freer, natural look. And remember to cut it only when it's dry. This works well for both girls and boys, although older boys are apt to resist a head of ringlets no matter how charming it looks to you.

To find someone who can cut your child's curls, follow the same advice I give to adults (see chapter 9, page 91) because not every hairdresser can cut curls. To trim your child's hair yourself, follow the tips in chapter 10 (see page 99). The trimming techniques are helpful if you just want to clean up their knotty, frayed ends or trim their bangs, which tend to need a cut sooner than the rest of their hair.

"When I was young, people used to ask me if my curls were a permanent. I would say, 'Yes, they are permanent—for life.'"
—LORRAINE

Baby Care

When my three kids were babies and I'd notice a dry patch on their scalps, I'd massage it gently with olive oil. After that, none of them had cradle cap (a yellowish crust that often develops on infant scalps), and their hair and scalps looked healthy and smelled clean. If your child does get cradle cap, both jojoba oil and olive oil are great for curing it. Gently rub the oil in the spot and leave it on overnight. In the morning, cleanse your child's hair with conditioner. (Extra virgin olive oil is also a great treatment for diaper rash!)

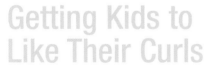

Getting Kids to Like Their Curls

I remember meeting a four-year-old girl whose father told me, "She hates her curls, so we try to point out women who have beautiful curly hair." The child had a head of gorgeous ringlets, but when I complimented her on them, she frowned and hid her head in her father's coat. It can be a casual remark made in the child's company, or perhaps someone making too much of a small

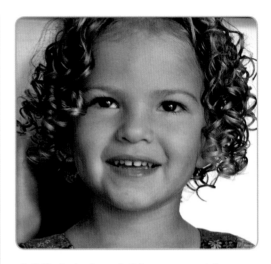

child's hair, but children are quick to pick up on prejudices of all kinds. Still, you can help them through it. Once in a while, point out a woman or man with beautiful curly hair. Or talk about how much you like your own curls. But don't make a big deal out of it or they'll figure something's up.

If you have naturally straight hair and your child has curly hair, find her a curly-haired mentor—someone she can bond with over her hair, its glory, its problems, and its orneriness. Many of us curly girls might have been spared years of agony, especially during adolescence, if only we'd had a curly-girl mentor to talk to. I'd spend hours in front of the mirror sobbing because I thought I looked hideous. When it was really humid, I'd run home during lunchtime and put on my brother's balaclava, a skin-tight woolen cap.

That's why I try to be a mentor to any curly haired child or teenager who needs it. I think my teenage years would have been very different if only an enlightened curly girl had taken me under her wing and said, "Call me if you have any questions about how to take care of your curls."

Note to Mom

If you are a curly girl who is still in denial of your curls and you have a curly kid, it's time to start loving your own curls. Whether you like it or not, you are your child's first beauty consultant. If you

curl confession

Asa Schiller *entrepreneur*

Being a curly girl married to a curly guy, I knew exactly how to handle my daughter Clara's curly hair. I've never straightened it or used a brush or shampoo, and I do a big conditioning once a week while she sits in the bath. This is very different from how my mother handled my curly hair. She'd brush it out, which hurt and made it look like a giant fuzz ball, and sigh, "I just can't do anything with this hair," which I interpreted as "your curls are ugly."

As an adult, I learned to just let my curls be. It's okay if a curl is sticking out on one side and if everything is not perfectly even. Once I realized this I felt such a huge sense of relief! I finally loved my curls and I wanted to pass this on to Clara from a young age. I wanted her to feel that having curly hair was

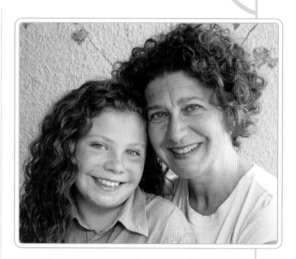

something unique and for her to feel good about her hair. People always compliment her curls (one woman said her hair made her look like a fairytale princess) and often say they love it. But they're not the only ones. Clara loves her hair. She sees it as special and beautiful. And if that doesn't warm a curly mom's heart, I don't know what does!

How to Gently Remove the Knots

■ **DO** saturate the knot and surrounding area with conditioner.

■ **DO** isolate the knot with one hand and hold it in between your thumb and forefinger. With the other hand, gently pry each strand of hair from the knot.

■ **DO** be gentle. Think of these knots as the equivalent of releasing a piece of jewelry that's gotten caught in your favorite sweater. You wouldn't tug and rip, you'd be ever so gentle when removing it.

■ **DON'T** use a brush or a comb, which will shred and pull hair and fuse the open cuticles that then attach to each other like Velcro.

■ **DON'T** attempt to remove knots without conditioner or you will break and rip the hair, which will cause more knotting in the near future.

love your curls, your child will love hers. But if you hide them—even if you never actually talk about not liking your curls, or you straighten your hair—you'll send a message that curls are something to hide and be ashamed of. So many of my curly clients recall mothers who did this, making them believe that straight hair was beautiful and curly hair was ugly.

Other women talk about not feeling accepted by their mothers because of their mothers' disdain of their curls. Comments like, "Oh, so that's how you wear your hair these days" or "Do something with your hair; it looks awful" hurt them so deeply

that memories of these remarks still sting even though some of these women are in their fifties!

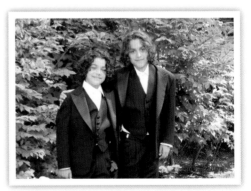

Shelley Ozkan's (page 31) boys take after their mom and wear their curls with pride.

curl confession

Sophie Portnoy *age fourteen*

When my wavy hair turned really curly in sixth and seventh grade, I started straightening it—a task that was totally exhausting. At 11 P.M., after studying and homework, I'd spend an hour and a half blowing it dry and flat-ironing it. Then I'd get into bed and try to sleep carefully so I wouldn't mess up my hard work. By morning, a few curls had escaped so I'd spend more time trying to iron them out.

One day, a friend asked me why I straightened my hair. When I told her it was because a boy I had a crush on said he liked it straight, she said, "If he really likes you, he'll like you whether your hair is straight or curly." She was right! So I put away my blow-dryer and flat iron and let my curls just be. They looked limp and unhealthy at first, but once I stopped torturing them, they began to look great. And that taught me a valuable lesson: I shouldn't straighten my hair—or do anything else in life—because of what someone else thinks.

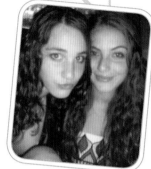

Sophie, left

Curls on the Verge

To put it mildly, puberty is a hormonal, sensitive time. Your child's face breaks out, his voice cracks, and she can go from smiling to sulking in the span of mere minutes. Then there's hair that starts to sprout everywhere! Plus, because of puberty, tweens and teens have overactive sebaceous glands, so hair tends to get oily and it can also change from soft and straight to coarse and curly. In fact, I've noticed that the hair of some of my young clients can change from one appointment to the next: It can get thicker, wavier, or curlier in a matter of months. Sometimes it's dry or frizzy, and other times lank and oily. I call these puberty curls or adolescent curls. (There are also times when, just by looking at a young client's hair, I can tell that puberty is just around the corner.)

My point in telling you this is to put you on alert. If your daughter breaks down sobbing because she can't manage her hair, she isn't just moody and dramatic. Her hair may very well be transforming from seemingly straight or wavy to curls and she has no clue about how to manage it. Your job is to guide her and help her understand and know how to care for her new hair. And if you can do that, at least one aspect of the teen years will be a bit easier.

Curly Cleansing 101

Once your child is old enough to shower alone, it's time for a quick course in curly cleansing. The earlier we teach our kids how to cleanse, condition, and style their hair, the better. When they're little, playfully explain to them what you're doing when you are cleansing and conditioning their locks during bath time. That way, you've already planted the seed for good hair habits.

I knew it was time for some hair coaching with my son when I noticed white blobs of conditioner in his curls when he got out of the shower. I had him put on his swimsuit and head back into the shower, and I coached him from the sidelines: "That's not enough conditioner. Use more! Move it around with your fingers. O.K., rinse. You missed a spot! Now scrunch!" It may not sound like much fun, but it honestly made a big difference. He now loves his full head of bright red, hydrated, defined curls.

PONYTAIL CAUTION

The too-tight ponytails that I often see on tweens and teens are a bad idea because they pull on the hairline. This tension can cause the hair to fall out and the hairline to recede. Instead, pull the hair back loosely. Also, if the hair is thick, air-dry it or use a hair dryer with a diffuser before you pull it back. Otherwise, if it's wet and in a ponytail all day, it can still be damp by evening, and mold and odors can set in.

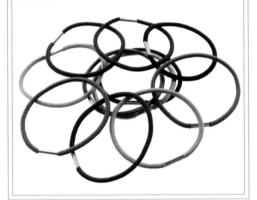

Take the time to teach your curly offspring the cleansing and care methods in this book. Just imagine that if we can teach the next curly generation the best way to care for their hair, we can change the world one gorgeous curl at a time. Then we can concentrate on other things like world peace!

curl confession

Clifton Green *professor at Emory University*

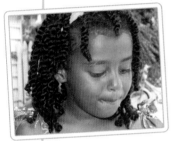

My adoptive daughter, Miriam, is black, while my wife and I are white. I'm the one who cares for her hair—an experience that has been filled with both joy and frustration and can take over an hour. After all, she's an active five year old so her hair is easily tangled. It's taken lots of discovery—we talked with other parents of multicultural kids and read lots of books—and practice. My twists and braids have come a long way but my cornrows still need work. I've realized that Miriam's hair is happier without daily washings, something that would make my hair greasy, and that I can use a fork to make her parts. Sometimes I make twists or braids; other days she wears it loose in

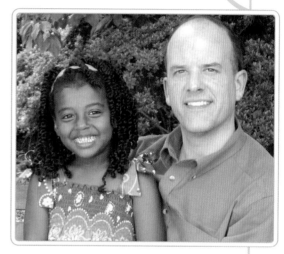

what we call "freedom" hair. I think of caring for her hair as laying the groundwork for when she's older and thinks about her identity as a woman of color. We're on the wait list to adopt another girl from Ethiopia so I'll have more chances to practice my skills!

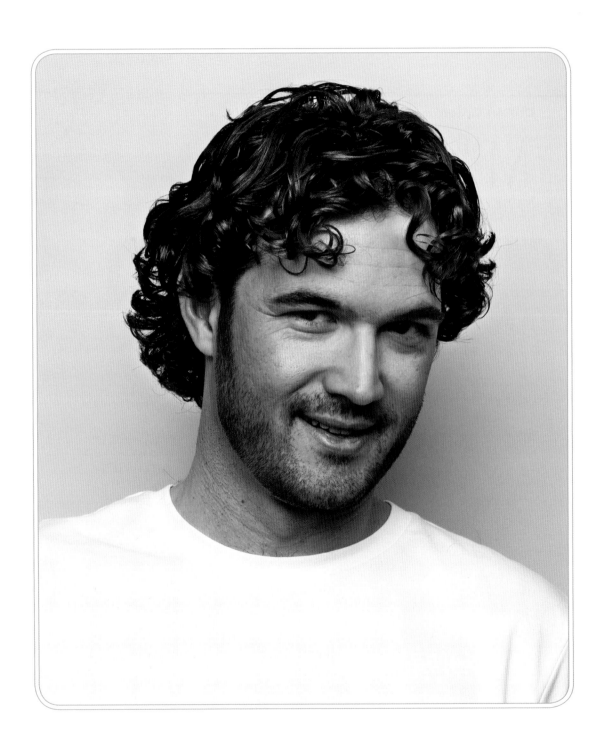

CHAPTER 13

guys 'n' curls

THE DOWN AND DIRTY ROOT-INE

Curls are a blessing not in disguise.

Since I wrote the first version of *Curly Girl*, I've been surprised that I've been hearing from the many curly guys out there. Sure, I knew there were many, many men with gorgeous curls, waves, and s'waves, but who knew they would pick up a book called *Curly Girl* and then take the time to write to the author? Well, they did. In droves! And they asked for their own chapter, so here it is.

Curly guys can simply follow the same routines as curly girls. But I know that most guys don't want to spend as much time on their hair as women do. So, I'm giving you a down-and-dirty routine with only the essential steps. If you are a curly guy, and you currently cleanse your hair and apply a styling product, your new curly hair routine won't take much longer than what you're doing now.

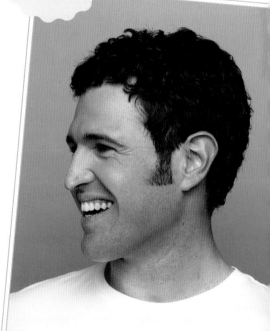

What's important is how and with what you cleanse your hair and the styling products you apply.

A lot of men use shampoo to clean their hair. But if you're a curly guy, what you need to use is either a 100-percent sulfate-free cleanser or a botanical conditioner to cleanse your hair. Most days, that's all you'll need to make your hair look great. The sulfate-free feature is key, because the chemicals in shampoos are damaging and drying to your hair and scalp. Since men are prone to rapid hair thinning and loss after the age of thirty, the last thing you want to do is subject your scalp and hair to chemicals that will only speed up the process.

Anecdotal evidence from many of our male clients and Devachan experts indicates that quitting their shampoo habit helped with their hair thinning and hair loss. Edward Fagley, Deva Color expert, was losing his hair before he came to work at the salon almost thirteen years ago. "I admit that I thought Lorraine was crazy when she suggested that clients never use shampoo," says Edward. "But once I stopped shampooing, I stopped losing my hair. The hair that I *do* have looks and feels fuller because the products I use fill it with moisture and give it natural volume." Going naturally curly also helps conceal thinning hair,

because curls' spherical shapes fill in space, making hair appear thicker than it really is.

Men often complain about dandruff. If you are one of them, you may be mistaking a simple dry scalp caused by harsh detergent-laden shampoos for a medical condition. Using shampoo to get rid of this supposed dandruff only clogs the pores, which turn into flakes, starting a vicious circle. Once you stop sudsing up your hair with detergents, your scalp will be healthier.

CURLY GUY ROOT-INE

THE DOWN-AND-DIRTY

Here are a few basic steps to make your hair look great:

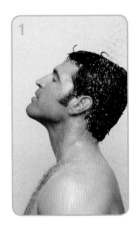

1 **Wet:** Step under the showerhead and let the water run through your curls. Resist the urge to start scrubbing your head; this disrupts your curls' basic shape. If you've got long hair, cup it in your hands so the water flow doesn't distort your curls' intrinsic pattern. Wet your hair thoroughly.

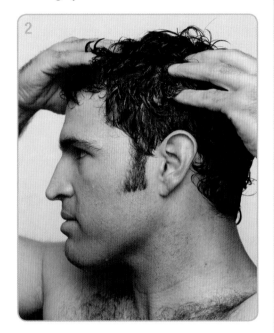

2 Cleanse: Apply either a sulfate-free cleanser or a botanical conditioner along your fingertips the way you'd apply toothpaste to a toothbrush, and evenly distribute it to your other fingertips. Then place your fingertips directly on the scalp, and using firm circular motions, massage the product into the scalp to stimulate blood flow, remove dirt particles, and keep your scalp healthy and hydrated. If your hair is long, apply an extra dollop of conditioner to the hair near the nape of

the neck, which tends to get knotted. Gently remove any knots with your fingers.

3 Rinse: If your hair tends to get frizzy, leave most of the cleanser or conditioner in by standing away from the shower flow and splashing just a few handfuls of water on your hair. This prevents all the cleanser/conditioner from being rinsed out and allows the hair to stay hydrated. (After a few days of rinsing your hair this way, you'll get a sense of how much rinse water your hair requires in order for you to be pleased with the outcome.)

4 Scrunch: Turn off the shower, lean forward, and scrunch your hair gently upward to remove some of the water and cleanser or conditioner.

5 Dry: Many men dry their hair by holding one end of a towel in each hand and rubbing it harshly over their head. But the rough fibers of the towel combined with this kind of friction causes hair to frizz. Instead, shake your head once or twice or use an old cotton T-shirt to scrunch the hair a bit so it's not dripping wet.

6 Style: Apply gel to your hands and scrunch it into your hair. How much gel you use depends on the length of your

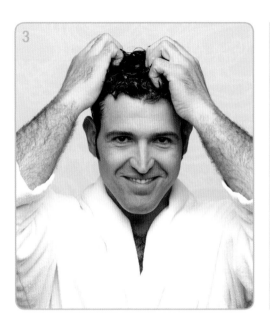

hair and how much hold you want (use more gel for more hold). Then let your curls air-dry so you don't cause frizz. Once your hair is totally dry, either leave it as is for a wet, contained look, or scrunch your hair gently to break the gel cast that has formed while the hair was drying.

Scrunch in the morning, then just walk away.

curl confession

Michael Graeser *health-care executive*

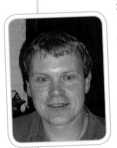

Growing up, everyone around me seemed to have hair that looked the same all the time, unlike my unpredictable wavy, curly hair that looked different each day. (It still does.) I often felt like a geek, wishing I had trendy, straight hair that would lie nice and flat instead of fluffy and all over the place. One year for yearbook photos, my hair was so supercurly that my photo sticks out from the other kids' photos like a stop sign.

About a year ago, I decided that I'd had enough of conforming to what other people wanted. I had to embrace my curly hair—and who I am—and let it do what it wanted. I gave up shampoo and brushes and started conditioning it often. I was blown away by the results. Everyone compliments me on my beautiful hair. Amazingly, ever since I decided to go curly, I've been happier and have more self-confidence than ever before. I finally feel like my life is coming full circle!

curl confession

Jordan Pacitti *professional dancer and fragrance company owner*

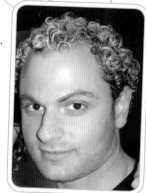

As a young child, my blond curls were soft, smooth, and defined, and people would rave about them. All that changed when I turned ten. The kids at school called me Brillo pad and said I had "caveman hair." On top of all of this, there weren't any hair idols to look up to at that age. So I just gave up. I kept my curls hidden with short haircuts and would brush them into submission—even though a wave always found its way out.

When I was fifteen years old, studying at the School of American Ballet in New York City, I was surrounded by people who were so individual that I realized I could let my curls out. I started growing my hair and mixing and matching products to see what would give me those beautiful curls. Also, around this time 'NSYNC was the most popular boy band and Justin Timberlake quickly became my hair idol. My hair looked good. Then I gave up shampoo, and my hair turned into the most amazing thing I could ever imagine.

CURLY GUY CUTS

A lot of curly guys have had their hair cut supershort for so long that they've forgotten they have curls. Like women who are chronic blow-dryers and flat-ironers, they will actually say, "I used to be curly!" But just because curls are mistreated doesn't mean they cease to exist. I have never witnessed curly hair going straight naturally—maybe looser but not straighter.

I've also heard a lot of short-haired men say, "But if I let my hair grow, my curls grow outward and I look like Bozo the Clown." It's true that back in the day of harsh shampoos and brushes, these curlies would tend to look like this favorite clown. But those days are gone and I assure you that growing out your curls on a diet of sulfate-free cleansing and conditioning products will prevent your hair from ballooning out atmospherically. In time, with length, gravity, and moisture, your hair will sprout and blossom into gorgeous, sexy curls.

One of the most important things is to find a stylist who understands curly hair and knows how to cut it, especially since guys get more frequent trims than girls. (See chapter 9, page 91, on finding a stylist to cut your hair, and ask him or her the questions on page 95.)

Here are some styles that look good on curly guys:

■ The hair style of D'Artagnan, one of the three musketeers in the Dumas classic, is a look that I would describe as unpretentious and sexy. It's not too long and not too short. It's worn just above the shoulders.

■ Caesar curls—or Roman curls—can also look stylish on men. You may have to skip two or three haircuts to allow your curls to grow past their first C shape (see page 93). This can be frustrating at first, but stick with it. Each time you feel the desire to cut your hair, imagine it setting you back to the hair you had three weeks earlier. If you really want to grow your hair, you just have to grow it! When my client Allesandro was trying to grow his hair, he came in for a trim twice and both times I turned him away. He was frustrated but I convinced him to stick with it, and now he has the long locks he never thought he could have, and he is delighted.

■ During the day for work, you can keep your hair in the gel cast to contain its girth and then open it up after work by scrunching your hair gently. Men with longer locks may want to wear bandannas or baseball caps when working out.

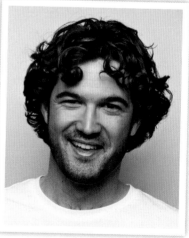

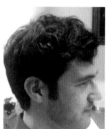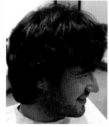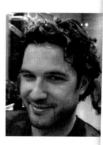

Allesandro grew out his hair from a short crop to the longer locks, right.

By being patient, Allesandro now has the long curly locks he wanted.

curl confession

Allen Salkin *investigative reporter*

I had gotten accustomed to being butchered. Envision it: I entered a salon, a barber shop, some place I thought my hair might have a chance of being safe. I did not want to be there, but my hair was unwieldy, demanding a trim. I pretended to be friendly to the person who greeted me, pasting a smile on my face, and then asking some inane question of the haircutter, like, "How long have you worked in this neighborhood?" I was like a prisoner trying to charm the person who is about to torture him, hoping that perhaps a bit of fake friendliness will entice the torturer to not break the prisoner's knuckles quite so unevenly this time. It was stupid, because I knew that it was extremely likely this person would do to me what all the other scissor wielders had done: cut and cut and reshape, and try to balance things out.

The haircutter would mutter: "Oh, I need to just clean that up." For them "clean that up" meant diving into my curls like a gardener with shears attacking an overgrown rhododendron. Snip snip. Hack, hack, hack. And there I'd be, feeling like 10 pounds had been cut off my head, a sort of pleasant feeling at first, an airy lightness, until I'd look in the mirror and see that this haircutter's version of cleaning things up was the same as all the others: hacking most of the curl out of my hair and getting down near scalp level.

It is hard to describe to someone who doesn't have curly hair what it is like to walk out of a salon and feel like all your power is gone, like someone has reached into your secret pouch of magic dust, pricked a hole in the bottom, and let the contents fall uselessly onto a dusty floor, where some minion will sweep it up like a bunch of poodle crap and throw it away with dirty cotton balls and half-eaten bananas. Poooof.

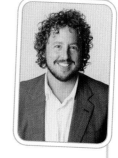

Listen, life isn't perfect. My stomach isn't the flattest. The stories I write sometimes get edited in ways that make me cringe. My neighbors sometimes cook things that smell awful. I'm not special in a lot of ways. But my hair is special. Somehow it expresses who I feel myself to truly be. It curls in strange double-helix coils like DNA, proud of its essence. It speaks. It lives. Sometimes when I'm down, the curls lie limply. Happy, and they bounce. And on those days when the wind dries my hair out and it flies in a jillion directions like straw ready to catch fire in a field, I will stop and realize something isn't right with my thinking about life. What do I need to change? Get it right, and the curls seem to regain their spring.

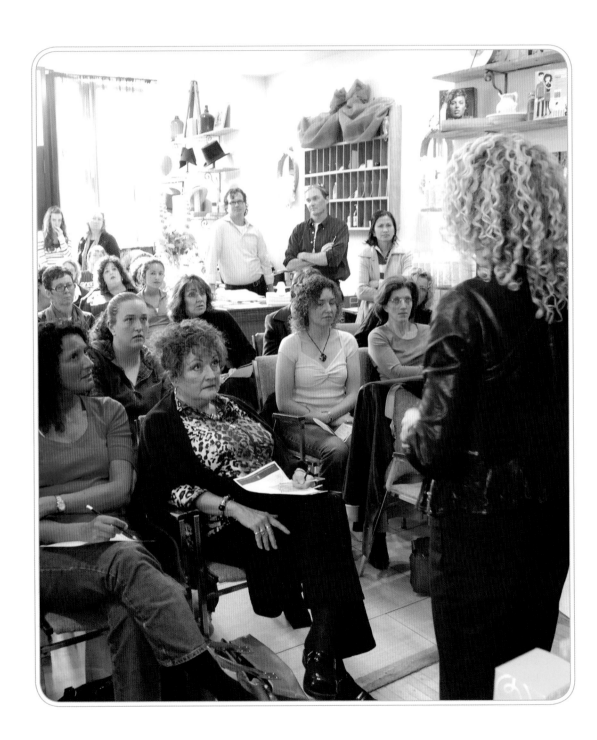

CHAPTER 14

curly Q's and A's

Q **Why doesn't the front of my hair grow as long as the back?**

cause and EFFECT

A The hair around your face, like the windshield of a car, is constantly exposed to wind, rain, heat, and other environmental factors, and therefore has a shorter life span than the rest of your hair. But you can mend and protect these tendrils by nurturing them with extra doses of conditioner and handling them gently. Pay attention to the damage you may be unwittingly inflicting on your hair by pulling it, playing with your bangs, or running your fingers through your locks.

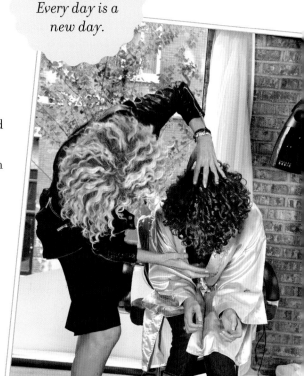

Accepting my curls is Zen: Every day is a new day.

How come my hair doesn't grow past a certain point?

Longing to Grow

Lots of curly girls complain about this. When you're using sulfate-filled shampoos, the ends of the hair get eroded and fray, stunting your hair's growth. Once you have weaned your strands off these damaging substances and your hair is hydrated again, it can and will start to grow.

How can I exercise and keep my curls looking great?

Work It Out

If you know you're going to cleanse your hair after a workout, simply tie it back at the nape of the neck or up at the crown with a fabric-covered ponytail holder, ribbon, or scarf. If you don't plan to shower after your workout and your bangs are short, either use a thin headband right at the front of your hairline to move the shorter pieces off your face (after the workout, this can give you a nice root lift, too) or twist the curls that frame your face back to the crown and anchor them with bobby pins. The twists will stop frizz and regenerate your hair's shape while harnessing it in place. Then gather the rest of your curls in a low or high ponytail, depending on your preference.

You can also try the Unicorn ponytail or the Samurai Bun (see pages 145–146).

How can I protect my curls while wearing a hat, bike helmet, or wig?

Protect + Revive

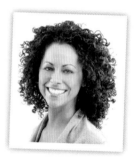

Curls have a cushioning nature and revive forgivingly with the right touch, especially those that are healthy and hydrated. So it's easy for your hair to recover from being compacted under a hat, hood, helmet, scarf, cap (like those worn by doctors and nurses), or a pair of earmuffs. In general, these things don't cause frizz, just flatness. And if the hair is positioned correctly beforehand, covering it can help set the hair and reduce frizz. Here's how:

1 Before putting on a hat or other head covering, apply gel directly to a clip or bobby pin, then place the clip or pin at the roots of the hair perpendicular to the scalp. A clip will keep the roots elevated while the weight of your head covering is pressing down on them.

2 If your hair is past shoulder length, gently gather it at the nape of the neck with a fabric-covered ponytail holder. Twist the curly tail upward and anchor it to the back of your head with bobby pins. If you have short curls around the front, take sections of these hairs and twist them backward toward the crown. This quick positioning of your curls will keep them in their natural formation, and they will regenerate when you set them free again.

3 When uncovering your hair, resist the urge to fluff it up. Instead, spritz it with lavender spray or wet your hands slightly under a running tap and place damp fingers at the roots. Tilt your head over and gently shuffle your fingertips to open the hair. Lift your hands off the scalp without running your fingers through your hair. Then scrunch the hair upward in the same manner that you scrunch gel when styling.

4 To give the top layer of hair more lift, lightly spritz a few of the flattened curls with lavender spray or water. Twist each section around your index finger, then slide the curl off and either pin or hold it in place with your fingers for a couple of minutes. (If water isn't available, just lick your finger to create the proverbial spit curl.)

How can I protect my curls while I sleep?

SLEEP-IN BEAUTY

Tossing and turning in bed at night causes a lot of friction. I suggest that you get a pillowcase made of silk, cotton sateen, or very high thread-count cotton to reduce friction and minimize split ends. The softer and more luxurious the cotton, the less damage it will do to your hair. You can also do one of the following:

■ **Sleep Like a Geisha:** Lie on your back and spread your hair over your pillow like you would spread out a veil. Just make sure to put a pillow right under your knees so you're in an ergonomic position with your nape and knees elevated. Sleeping on your back also prevents the hair on the side you sleep on from becoming weaker than the hair on the other side.

■ **The Unicorn:** Bend forward at the waist and tilt your head forward. Gather your hair gently at the center of the forehead with a fabric-covered ponytail holder, ribbon, or scarf. If

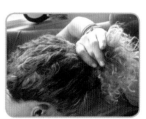
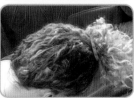

your hair is really curly, pull it through so it's free flowing. The Unicorn prevents the ends of your hair and the curls at the nape of the neck from getting knotted, and also prevents frizz if it rains during the night. The next morning, remove the ponytail holder. Spritz the hair with lavender spray or wet your hands slightly, place your fingertips gently on your scalp, and lightly shuffle hair at the roots. Then let your hair settle. This process will loosen the curls at the nape without disfiguring them, and they will appear longer the next day.

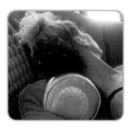

■ **The Samurai Bun:** Tilt your head forward and gather your hair at the crown using a fabric-covered ponytail holder. As you loop the band the second or third time, don't pull the hair through, so it resembles a fan. As with the Unicorn, when you let down your hair, use your fingertips to lightly shuffle the hair at the roots. Then decide whether it needs a full-on cleansing or just a spritz with lavender spray.

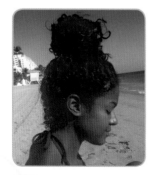

The Samurai Bun

What can I do for an itchy scalp?

IF YOU HAVE AN ITCH, SCRATCH IT

If you're recovering from a long-term addiction to shampoo, your scalp will probably be going through an adjustment period. It's like weaning yourself off bubbly sodas and replacing them with carrot juice. An itch is often a sign that your scalp is healing, like a scab itches as a wound begins to heal. It's also a sign that your scalp needs more moisture. After all, shampoo abuse has kept the scalp (and your curls) in a constant state of dehydration. For immediate relief, whip up the exfoliating scalp scrub (see page 84). Wet your hair thoroughly, and apply the scrub to your scalp using circular, massaging motions. Rinse hair thoroughly, and condition it. Also, try spot-cleansing (see page 42) or spritzing your scalp with lavender spray (see page 83), which contains natural medicinal properties that help soothe and cleanse the skin.

If the itching continues, you may have a scalp condition, so see your doctor. Remember, however, that some doctor-recommended prescriptions may heal the scalp but can wreak havoc on the hair. If you need to use a prescribed product, first apply a generous amount of botanical conditioner to wet hair. Then, and only then, apply the doctor-recommended product to the scalp. That way, when you're rinsing out the harsh topical prescription, the barrier of conditioner is protecting your precious locks. What a difference this simple solution makes to the preservation of your hair!

My color grows out so fast and my roots look like a landing strip! Any suggestions?

Escape ROOTS

When your curls are wet or dry, take a bobby pin that's close to the color of your hair and apply gel to it. Weave the bobby pin through the roots of the hair, taking strands from each side of your part as though you're sewing a seam together. Once the hair is dry, the hairpin will have given your hair a lift and it will hide your roots. You can either leave the bobby pin in or take it out.

In a pinch and for the short-term, you can use "hair mascara" (any waterproof mascara will do) to touch up your roots.

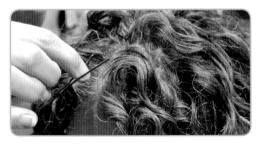

I'm having a bad hair day. Help!

No more BaD HaIr Daze

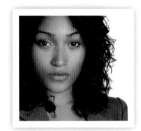

Certainly some days are *hairier* than others. Maybe you're rushing off first thing on a morning when you didn't put enough conditioner or gel in your hair and a strong gust of wind disturbs your well-defined curls. Or you go shopping, try on lots of sweaters, and leave the dressing room with your hair flying out in all directions. What can you do short of grabbing a hat or pulling those curls back in a ponytail?

Spritz your hair with water or lavender spray. Then wind a few curls tightly around your finger, and clip them for a minute or two to recreate your bouncy, defined curl. Or tilt your head so that your hair falls forward, place your fingertips on your scalp, and give the roots a shuffle to lift and open the hair. One thing to note: You're a curly girl, so even if your hair isn't behaving the way you want it to, you may be the only one who knows it! Own it and accept all that it gives you.

My hair looks dull. How can I get it to shine?

GLISTEN TO ME

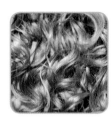

Shine is always an issue with curly hair. Unlike straight hair, which has a flat surface and can reflect a lot of light, curly strands have contours so light reflects only off part of them. Also, if your hair's past includes shampooing, blow-frying, and straightening, be patient. You may never get the sheen that your naturally straight sisters can achieve, but after a few weeks of TLC and conditioner, conditioner, and more conditioner, shinier curls will emerge.

I'm going through menopause. Can the hot flashes and night sweats negatively affect my hair?

THE PLUSES TO THE FLUSHES

Actually, curly hair can benefit from the extra moisture that you're suddenly producing. Sweat is part of the body's ecosystem and is a natural cleansing agent. If the hot flashes are especially frequent or severe, you may want to wear your hair up (see chapter 15, page 156, for updos), especially in situations when you feel the need to keep your cool. Or try a shorter hairstyle. And always carry a travel size bottle of lavender spray in your bag for a refreshing spritz to your hair, face, or neck when you're on the go.

My hair sometimes looks stringy, not curly. Is this from too much product?

GRANOLAS, NOT CURLS, ARE SUPPOSED TO CRUNCH

Overcleansing and leaving in too much conditioner or using alcohol-filled gels can give the hair a petrified, wet, crunchy look. It doesn't allow the hair to swell to its natural, three-dimensional girth. If you're cleansing daily, give hair a break and just refresh with a spritz of lavender spray at the roots. Brushing and combing can also cause frayed, stringy strands, so toss that brush and simply use your fingers to comb through your hair in the shower when it's slathered in conditioner. The other message your stringy strands may be sending is that it's time for a trim or possibly a shape change.

Q I'm really short on time in the morning. Do I need to wet my hair every day?

IF IT AIN'T Broke, DON'T FIX IT

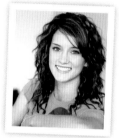

A Your hair will tell you whether it needs a full-on cleansing to look and feel its best. Some curly girls report that cleansing or wetting their hair once every three days is all they need; others need to cleanse more often. You be the judge. If you don't have time for even a quick spritz or a clip at the roots in the morning, you may want to reevaluate your schedule—and what really matters to you.

Q What is a clarifying shampoo, and does it restore shine?

Packaging, Packaging

A Let me clarify one thing. I have no faith in shampoos, and those that say "clarifying" terrify me even more. Products such as après-pool shampoos or clarifying shampoos and conditioners are merely another way to sell you more of what you don't need. These products are often harsher on hair than regular shampoos, stripping it of hydration. Don't waste your money on one more cleverly packaged product that will probably damage your hair and make your curls look worse! Just keep up your new, curly girl routines.

Q I travel a lot. How do I protect my hair from changes in climate and water?

Wherever you go, you Take your curls

A Your hair is a natural weather barometer, so trust what it tells you. Though there's no need to adjust your hair care routine, you may have to vary the amount of conditioner you leave in the hair and the amount of gel you use on your traveling locks. You may find that you need less in Los Angeles because the weather is generally dry—a perfect climate for curls—and more in England where frequent drizzle can bring out the frizzies in even the best-tressed curls. Don't leave home without your conditioner and lavender spray: Both will see you through almost any climatic situation. (And the moisturizing spritz is great for refreshing your skin, hair, or other body part midflight.)

My jet-set trick is to cleanse and condition my hair the morning of the flight and scrunch in more gel than usual. Then I let it set in its gel cast for the duration of the flight so I can sleep or fidget for hours and still have frizz-free, moist curls on arrival. When it's time to land, I tilt my head forward, shake it at the roots, and then gently scrunch upward to dissolve the gel cast and open hair to reveal bouncy jet-set curls.

How do I avoid a bad case of the frizzies?

Frizz is a dirty word

Frizz is a curl waiting to happen. Sometimes it's shampooed hair begging for moisture (its natural survival requirement). But here's how you can defrizz:

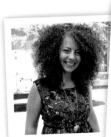

Before

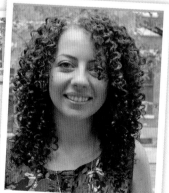

After

▦ On rainy or high-humidity days, wet hair thoroughly and use extra conditioner to help elongate your hair so it goes in a north-south direction instead of an east-west one (see page 30).

▦ Don't linger too long in a steamy bathroom after showering. The humidity can open up the hair's cuticle, causing a high frizz factor.

▦ Another frizz-buster is giving curls one last cool rinse to seal the cuticle before styling. Fill a bowl with cool water, and if you're really determined, put ice in it. Then dunk your hair in after you get out of the shower. Tilt forward, and with your hands scrunch out as much of the water and conditioner as you can. Then scrunch a palmful of gel in the hair, and when bringing your head to an upright position, graze extra gel or spray-gel on the canopy in a downward motion to keep the cuticle smooth.

▦ Don't touch your hair once you've applied gel, no matter how tempted you are to pat the strands into place. This general rule for curly girls is particularly important on frizz-prone days.

▦ If you have a special occasion like a prom or a date, here's how you can protect your locks and encourage your curls to swell to their natural state with absolutely no frizz. After cleansing and styling (as discussed above), spritz spray gel onto a silk scarf and loosely lay it over your hair. Clip the scarf at the back of your head and leave it on for 5 to 10 minutes. The scarf acts as a light weight that won't allow the cuticle on the canopy of the hair to rise.

One more thought on the subject of frizz: It is not necessarily a bad thing. I personally like my halo at times, and I have clients who feel the same way. I think that if hair is healthy and the curls are basically well defined, a slight halo can be appealing. In fact, I've received many compliments on days when I haven't fought the frizz too much. (Maybe I'm the only one who sees it!) I have long accepted frizz as one of the ways in which my curls choose to express themselves.

How can I get rid of static?

Hair-raiser!

Most curly girls don't have much of a static problem once they throw away the hairbrush, shampoo, and harsh electric appliances that create static blow-fly!

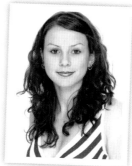

Use plenty of conditioner, especially on the canopy of the hair. If static and flyaways are still a problem, take a wet paper towel with gel in it, and graze gently in a downward motion over the top layer of your hair.

Tied in a knot

Tie your curls back *with* your curls. To get your hair off your face or for end-of-the-day droop, try this pretty solution.

First, pull your hair back. Take a 1-inch section of hair from behind each ear. Cross the two strands over the rest of your hair and tie. Then pull a couple of curls out around the front to frame your face. For more on this look, see page 172.

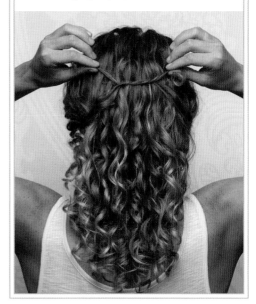

Q

Why do I have knots at the nape of my neck?

WHAT Knots?

A

If you're a breathing human being living in constant movement, accept the knots to be a part of daily life whether you're curly or knot. I call it the maypole effect, when hair strands, which are falling off the head on a curved but fixed axis, spin when the head moves. To gently remove the knots, saturate them and surrounding hair with a botanical conditioner, which will prevent the hair from breaking and ripping. With one hand, isolate the knot and hold it between the thumb and forefinger. With the other hand, gently pry and release each strand of hair from the knot. Do not shred or pull, or you will fuse the open cuticle.

Q

Why do my ends become much drier and more brittle in the winter?

HAPPY ENDINGS

A

If your locks are shoulder length or longer, the ends are apt to be drier because your hair is constantly

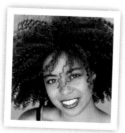

rubbing against the rough texture of fabrics like wool, coat collars, and scarves. (In the summer, there's less friction with light, smooth fabrics.) There is not much you can do other than hypercondition and seal the ends with a silicone-free, alcohol-free product. And remember to gently remove any trapped hair out from under your coat, scarf, or bag handle! Also, try a late-winter trim.

Q

Will it ever be possible for me to have bangs?

FRINGE BENEFITS

A

Actually, it is possible to have funky, cropped bangs as long as you realize that they will never lie flat. Take two or three dry curls over your forehead, and have them cut shorter to frame and soften your face. Make sure they're cut when the hair is dry (never wet), and don't have them cut straight across. On days when your bangs simply won't behave or they spring back too much, keep them weighted while the hair is drying by placing a clip at the end of each wayward curl. You can also create faux bangs with freshly cleansed and well-gelled hair. Just place clips at the concave bend of each wave to hold it in place as it dries, or if the hair is not newly cleansed, spray it with water or a spray gel and then clip. This timeless romantic look "alludes" to bangs, similar to Rita Hayworth's bangs, without committing to real ones.

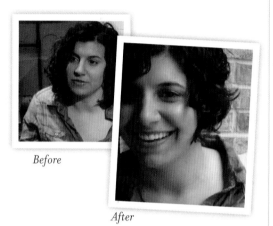

Before

After

May I ever blow-dry my hair?

CURL, INTERRUPTED

No, because even one blow-fry can set you back. But if the weather is frigid and you're in a rush to leave the house, you can use a blow-dryer with a diffuser on low to medium heat or a free-standing hooded dryer. I dry my curls by turning on the heat in my car, which creates a little microclimate that allows the moisture from the products to lock into the hair faster, keeps the hair cuticle closed, and evaporates the water.

What's the best way to tie back my curly hair or put it in a ponytail without causing breakage?

TIE ME UP, TIE ME DOWN

Use a fabric-covered ponytail holder, hair sticks or chopsticks, bobby pins, or a leather-covered clasp held in place with wooden sticks. You could stylishly use your own hair to put it back (see page 151). Never use rubber bands or any other kind of elastic with a closed metal clasp that can pinch, gnaw, and saw on your hair as your head moves back and forth. Also, make sure you don't pull your ponytail back too tightly or your hairline will begin to recede.

I know I have to give up my blow-frying and shampoo habits, but I'm afraid that if I go natural, my hair will look terrible. How long will it take before my curls start to look good?

ADDICTED TO GADGETS

If your hair is wavy, you'll see more curls within three weeks; if you have Botticelli or corkscrew curls, it will take less time to notice a difference in definition. Although your hair will love going natural, you may need some time to get used to your new look. "Everyone loves my newfound curls, but I am having an identity crisis!" is a typical in-recovery statement. Just take it one day at a time, learn what your curls want, not what you want, and seek to coexist in the hair and now. Your curls will look great even if they don't conform to your exact vision. (Remember, your eyes have to adjust, too!) Abandon all the negatives and focus on the positives. Don't compare your hair with others'!

Q **What's the best way to protect my hair when swimming in the pool or ocean?**

swim-in-love

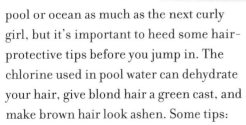

A I love splashing around in the pool or ocean as much as the next curly girl, but it's important to heed some hair-protective tips before you jump in. The chlorine used in pool water can dehydrate your hair, give blond hair a green cast, and make brown hair look ashen. Some tips:

■ Before swimming, pour extra virgin olive oil in your hands, rub them together, and apply in a downward motion to the top layer of your hair. How much you use depends on how dense your hair is. Since oil and water don't mix, the oil will repel the chlorinated water. Get a spray bottle from a hardware store to make applying the oil easier.

■ If you wear a bathing cap, spray the lining of the cap with olive oil. This not only protects the hair from breakage, but makes it easier to remove the cap after your swim.

■ *Never* use shampoo to wash your hair after swimming. The combination of chlorine and sulfates in shampoo adds a double dose of chemicals to your hair's delicate surface. And don't be fooled by products that promote themselves as "swimmer's shampoo," because most of these also contain sulfates. To remove chlorine, cleanse hair right after swimming with a sulfate-free cleanser or botanical conditioner and rinse. Apply another application of conditioner, comb it through with your fingers, and either leave it all in if you are sitting poolside or beachside or do a trickle rinse. (For those with very fine or straight hair, rinse out conditioner completely.) If you're unable to rinse your hair immediately after swimming, bring conditioner in a spray bottle to the pool and spritz it on hair each time you get out of the water.

Q I've been sick, depressed, on antibiotics, and broke up with my boyfriend. My hair looks awful. Is there a connection?

SPRING IS IN THE HAIR

A Any of those situations, individually or in combination, can have a profound effect on your curls. As a nonessential organ, your hair is at the bottom of the physiologic hierarchy, so it's likely to be neglected by the body when the immune system is fighting disease or depression. Even the mildest medications may have side effects, and your hair is not immune to these reactions. (One client swears that when she takes decongestants for a day or two, her normally bouncy curls get dry and flat.)

An emotional crisis or period of high stress can trigger skin conditions like acne, eczema, hives, psoriasis, and cold sores. So it's no surprise when your scalp and hair also reflect your emotional state. If you lose your job or are suffering from a break-up, you're likely to eat badly, stay up too late, and lie in bed instead of exercising, and your hair will reflect this. (And serious stress can also cause hair loss.) The good news is: Your hair will bounce back as soon as you do. In the meantime, keep it tied back lightly, don't skimp on conditioner, drink plenty of water, take a tablespoon of flax oil, fish oil, or olive oil, and, above all, don't make any drastic changes in your hairstyle. Wait until you're on the mend to experiment with a new cut or a different color.

BOYS WHO LOVE CURLS

Last year on an episode of the dating show *The Millionaire Matchmaker*, the matchmaker told a group of single, curly haired women to straighten their curls. "Men don't like curly hair," she said. I couldn't agree less! So I sought insight from men who love curls. Here's what a few had to say:

"My girlfriend is not as spontaneous when she straightens her hair! Her spirit goes away when her curls do! I love her the best when she's curly!"
—JASON, Australia

"There is nothing better than rolling over in the middle of the night to spoon your wife and nuzzle her curly curls."
—JOHN KNEISLEY

"Curly in the head, curly in the bed!"
—JEREMY HORN

"Curls are a truth serum. When she straightens her hair, I feel like she's hiding more than her hair."
—TODD, New York City

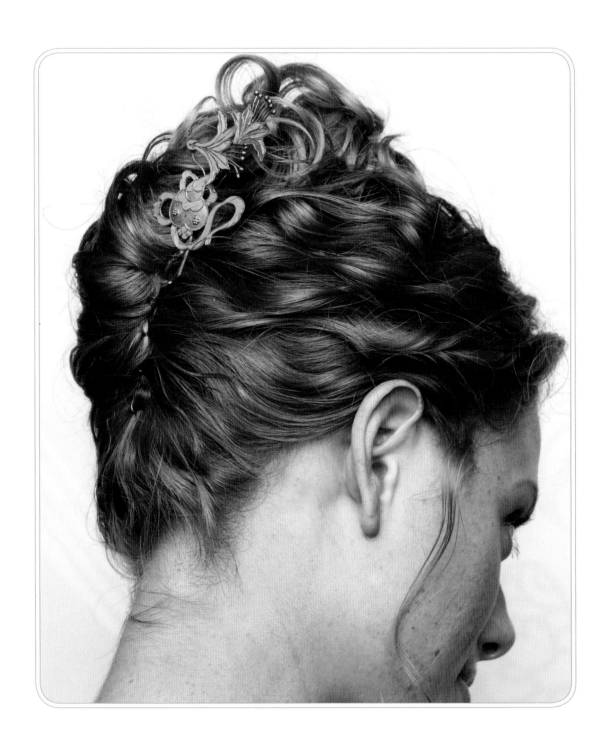

CHAPTER 15

wed-locks and updos for special occasions

I t's a fact that curly hair is different every day—sometimes every hour. Its unpredictable nature is probably why so many curly girls think blow-drying their precious curls straight is a good "social security" policy for big occasions. To tame Miss-behaving curls before becoming a Mrs., curly girls will even schedule their weddings based on seasons and geography, usually choosing autumn or winter in a very dry climate because of the lower humidity levels.

Some curlies will straighten their curls and then use a curling iron to mimic what their hair does naturally! (That's like replacing a natural food with a synthetic product that's been enriched with vitamins.) Then these curly girls use enough hair spray to burn a hole in the ozone and make their hair as hard as a Darth Vader helmet. I remember being at one wedding on a wet, rainy evening watching a sea of blow-outs—including the bride's—unfurl in front of me, every one of their dried out cuticles opening up, reaching out to the atmosphere, looking for moisture with their natural survival instinct. (I would do the same if I were in a dry desert!)

For most special occasions—and of course "the big day"—a lot of curly girls tell me they want to do something different with their hair, but want to look like themselves and not overdone. There are many individual, elegant updos you can create that allow your curls to be the star of the show and only require that you use what you already have. It's as simple as collecting your curls upward and pinning them gracefully next to each other. The first rule in any updo is to not overdo. If a few random ringlets fall out, leave them; all curly updos should make you look and feel like a goddess. Dressy barrettes, covered clips, broaches or necklaces made into hair jewelry, gold- or silver-colored threads or ribbons intertwined with your updo will certainly create tresses to impress.

On the big day, wake early to cleanse and set your hair as described for your curl type (see chapter 3, page 19), but use or leave in a bit more conditioner and gel to ensure no frizz (which can happen from touching your hair while you style). Don't start creating your updo until your hair is completely dry (except for the sleek Yin Yang look on page 169), which means you may have to get up extra early to give hair enough time to dry. Handle your curls gently and use a fabric-covered ponytail holder to prevent breakage. Whenever you wear a ponytail for a date, make it special by wrapping a piece of hair around the ponytail holder and secure it with a pin. Also important: Practice creating your wedding updo and the timing of it a couple of weeks or days before the special event.

Now, here's how to create twelve special-occasion looks that are sexy, playful, funky, elegant, and, best of all, easy to do yourself.

Goddess Curl

For long-haired girls with corkscrew curls, this updo will make you look like a goddess.

1 Gather your curls at the nape of the neck, and twist the hair gently while moving it in an upward direction. Roll the twist inward up the back of your head, stopping at the crown. This creates a seam or crease in the back.

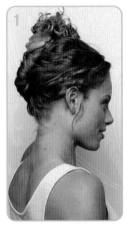

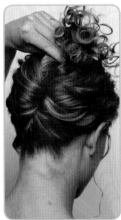

2 When you've twisted the strands as far as they will reach, hold your hair in place with one hand. With your free hand, secure the twist by weaving and inserting bobby pins into and along the seam.

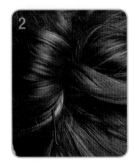

3 To soften the look, leave out a few strands around the hairline before putting your hair up.

4 If you have short hair, follow the instructions above, but make the twist very tight, and use as many bobby pins as you need to secure the shorter strands of hair. An exaggerated amount of exposed bobby pins can look really chic.

Crown 'n' Glory

For a romantic twist on the Goddess Curl updo, left:

1 Twist a strand of colored ribbon, leather, or a necklace, and place it on your head by crisscrossing it twice around the updo or chignon.

2 Pin the ribbon in place with bobby pins or tiny sequined clips, leaving any excess fabric or piece of jewelry to hang free at the nape. Or dress up your twist by inserting hair jewelry or a fresh flower at the side or intertwined in a curl or the seam of the chignon.

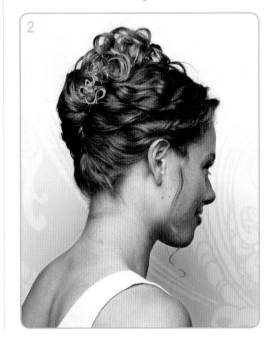

Curl Siren

With hair swept elegantly off to one side, this look is reminiscent of a retro '50s movie siren.

1 For this asymmetrical look, gather your hair to one side of your head so it rests at the shoulder.

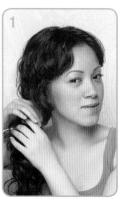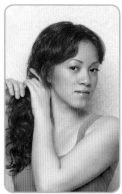

2 Loosely tie the hair with a ponytail holder.

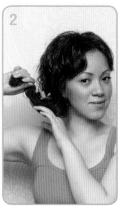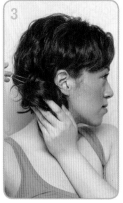

3 With four fingers, roll the ponytail backward, and anchor bobby pins in the seam of the roll.

4 Add a flower or another adornment for a special effect.

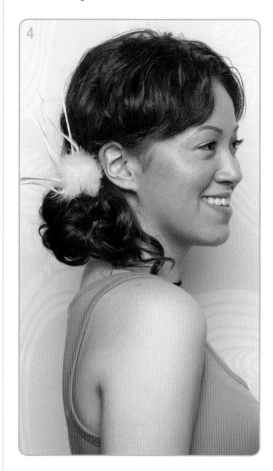

5 If the hair is shorter than the model's hair, above, just tie it and leave the curls to spring out loosely.

Long'n for Short

If you have long buoyant curls and want to make them appear shorter without forfeiting any length, here's what to do:

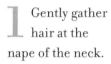

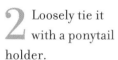

1 Gently gather hair at the nape of the neck.

2 Loosely tie it with a ponytail holder.

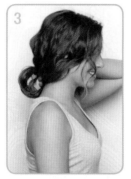

3 Roll the tail under to whatever length you prefer.

4 Tuck it under the nape and anchor it with four bobby pins.

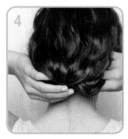

5 If you have shorter tendrils at the front, leave them out so hair looks like a bob or loosely twist them back and intertwine them into the shape.

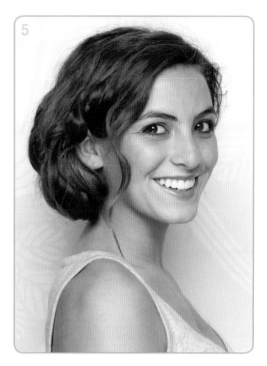

Warning: This updo look may give friends and family a shock, because they'll think you cut off your locks without consulting them first!

Sew Beautiful

Before bobby pins were invented, it was believed that the Elizabethans sewed their hair into place. This might be a good idea for you, too, if you have really thick, heavy hair that doesn't hold bobby pins during a night of dancing. All you need is a child's plastic sewing or embroidery needle and a piece of ribbon, thread, leather, wool yarn, or even fishing wire about 12 inches long.

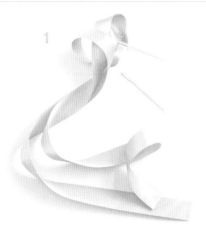

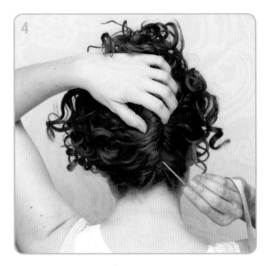

1 Thread the ribbon through the sewing needle.

2 Gather your hair at the nape of the neck.

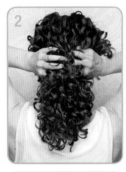

3 Hold the gathered hair with one hand, and using the other hand, take the loose part of the hair and begin twisting it upward until there's no more hair to twist (like in the Goddess Curl on page 158). Switch hands.

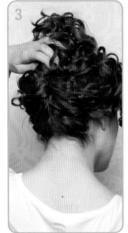

4 While one hand is holding the twisted hair, take the threaded sewing needle and, starting at the bottom, loop the ribbon through the seam of the twist as though you are sewing the hair together, and repeat until you reach the top of the seam.

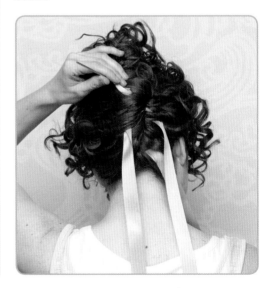

5 When all the ribbon is woven in, hide the needle inside the hair (optional) until you are ready to take your hair down.

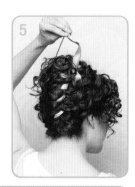

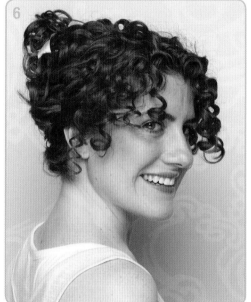

6 Loosen some tendrils in the front to frame the face.

7 You can embellish this updo by adding things like crystals and semiprecious stones (with loops on them so you can thread the ribbon through) intertwined through the hair.

Curl-Hawk

This is a fun and funky adaptation of the popular faux-hawk look, without the commitment.

1 Take a wide section of curls on the middle top of your head (from the forehead to the crown) and separate it out. Tie the hair at the back with a ponytail holder, wrap a strand of hair around the ponytail holder, and secure with a bobby pin. Gather the curls on top together loosely.

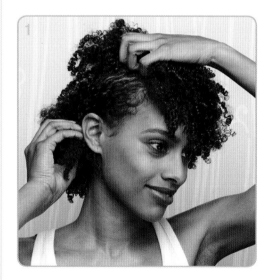

2 Spritz the remaining hair on both sides with spray gel, wetting it enough to make it look sleek when it's gathered at the back of the neck.

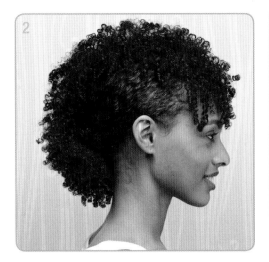

3 Twist it upward to the crown, and anchor it with bobby pins. If your top hair is short, let it go free and shake it at the roots to make it bigger. The two textures of the smooth hair at the sides and the curly hair up top can be as classy or wild as you like.

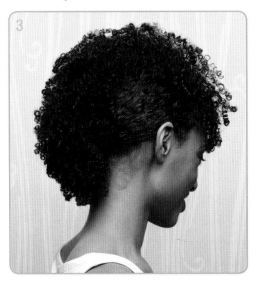

All Tressed Up...

. . . and know where to go. This "do" can be tressed down or tressed up by adding a hair adornment such as intertwined necklaces.

1 With your fingers, loosely part the hair from the crown to just behind the ear on each side of your head.

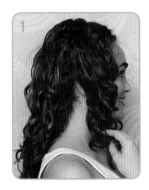

2 Gather the rest of your hair between the parted sections into a high ponytail and tie with holder. Wrap a piece of hair around the holder to hide it, and secure with a bobby pin.

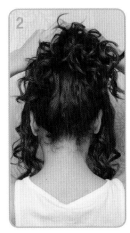
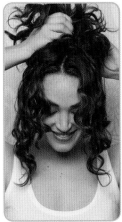

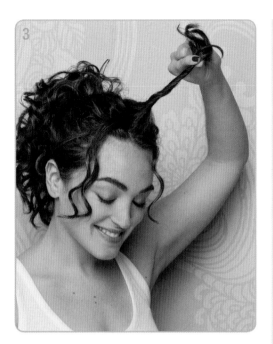

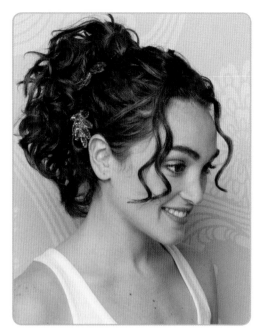

3 Take 1- to 2-inch–wide pieces of hair or individual defined curl sections and twist them back toward the ponytail and anchor with bobby pins. Twist separate sections of the remaining tendrils back in a random pattern around the central ponytail and anchor. Use a mirror to see the placement of your twists from the side and back. (Really thick hair may need two pins per twist.)

Adornments such as brooches and odd earrings can add sparkle to the do.

Some variations on this updo:

■ Braid one or more sections of tendrils instead of twisting.

■ Loop and weave one section under another one that is already anchored.

■ With wavy, s'wavy, and very long hair, take loose sections of the ponytail, spritz with spray gel, and lightly wrap them around your finger like a pin curl. Secure them with bobby pins. You can vary the size of these curls, making some small coils (by wrapping hair around one or two fingers) and others thicker (by wrapping around three or four fingers).

curl confession

Ellen Warren Chicago Tribune *columnist and senior correspondent*

As a tiny girl, my very first memories are of my hair—dry, frizzy, horrid. I wanted a long swishing ponytail. I got a pathetic puff ball. In middle school, the solution I settled on was a $1 military salvage store sailor's cap. With the brim pulled down, it became my trademark as I abandoned hope and just did the best I could to cover up my natural Brillo. At sixteen, I saved enough from my summer job to buy a wig made of human hair. It was not as straight (or as long) as the kind of hair I envied and it cost $250, a huge amount for a kid making only a few bucks an hour. But I lived in that wig, especially at the beach where salt air was toxic to a curly girl who wanted to sling her hair around like the women in the shampoo commercials. Wearing my wig as my high-school girlfriends and I walked the Rehoboth Beach boardwalk in Delaware, trolling for cute guys, I felt almost normal.

Ellen Warren's column caricature

In college, the discovery of inexpensive ($30) synthetic wigs was a breakthrough and a salvation. I bought several and had them professionally cut by a really good stylist. It was uncomfortable (and lumpy) to shove my thick, curly hair under a very tight wig, but that was a small price to pay for straight hair.

One memorable hair event transpired in a Maine lobster restaurant, where I was eating with some reporter friends after a day of covering President George H. W. Bush at his summer retreat in Kennebunkport. Joking around, one of the newsmen snatched the baseball cap off my head—and found himself also holding my "hair." I'd had a fake ponytail sewn onto the cap. The look on his face was priceless.

Fast-forward a decade, and I was working at the *Chicago Tribune*. I spotted a copy of *Curly Girl* at the office and paged through it. I told a colleague that I'd be the hair model if she decided to write about the author. She took me up on it, and when Lorraine came to Chicago, my curls got her personal attention.

From that experience, I knew that I needed to go to New York and have her work the full treatment on my horrible hair. After just one appointment, I felt that I had some control over the situation—something I'd never felt before. It changed my life.

Wrap-unzel

A playful twist and wrap updo by day. In the evening, unfurl the wrap and shake out to full, bouncy curls.

1 Gently pull your hair back into a low ponytail. For a soft look, leave out a few pieces of defined curls around your face; for a sleek look, gather all of the hair together at the nape.

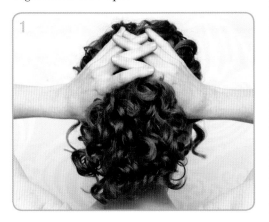

2 Wrap a ponytail holder around the hair two or three times, but don't pull the ponytail all the way through (you'll have some hair that is tucked in and some that will fall out).

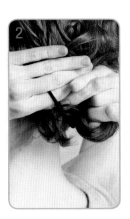

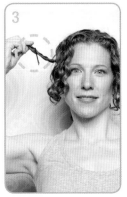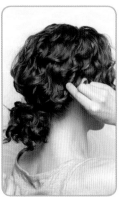

3 Loosely twist any front pieces of hair back. For best results, bring them forward so you can see them in the mirror, and place a bobby pin where you'll pin them, then bring the hair back and anchor it near the ponytail.

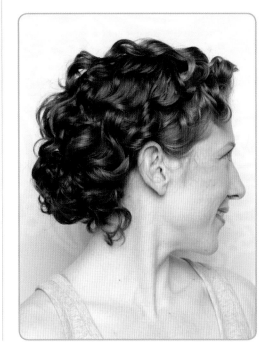

curl confession

Claire Warren *family physician*

There's a photo of me when I was two years old and my sister, Ellen (see page 166), was eight. We both had giant heads of crazy, curly hair. Everyone thought we looked adorable—everyone but us. We thought we looked ugly. Our childhood was the saga of the curly hair. We used cut-up orange juice cans as rollers and slept on them. We'd fry our hair by ironing it with a real iron and using wax paper to get it really shiny. Or we'd spend hours blow-drying it. Amazingly, in medical school I had no time for anything, but the little free time I *did* have, I'd spend drying my hair. I could get it straight, but the minute it rained or became humid, it went curly.

Then one day my sister called and told me about the Curly Girl religion and how you don't use shampoo or brush your hair. I didn't believe it until I saw Ellen's hair! It looked incredible. I got my hair cut and followed the Curly Girl Method. I was stunned, but my fuzzy curls became little ringlets. Today, people in the street stop me all the time to ask about my curls. Before I let them in on my secret, I say, "This conversation is going to change your life," because that's what happened to me. I'm

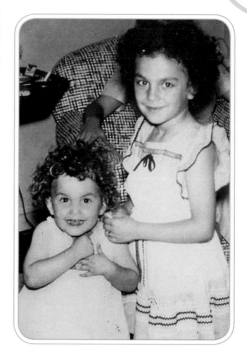

involved in a charter school where I met an African American girl whose hair was plastered against her skull. I shared with her what I did with my curls, and when I saw her a month and a half later, she had the most beautiful curls and the biggest smile on her face. It was like she was free!

Yin Yang Curls

The opposite textures of pulled-back sleek on top and curly ponytail behind are what give this hairdo its name.

1 Cleanse hair as described for your hair type in chapter 4, 5, or 6, leaving in more conditioner than you normally do.

2 While the hair is wet, smooth the top down with your fingers, making it as sleek as you can. Then bring it to the back into either a high ponytail or a low one at the center of the nape. (Usually, I don't recommend tight ponytails since they can cause your hairline to recede, but it's okay to do it once in a while for a special occasion.)

3 Take a piece of hair from your ponytail, braid it, and then wrap it around the ponytail holder and secure with a bobby pin. Scrunch loose hair in the ponytail upward and apply gel. Either diffuse the hair or allow it to dry naturally. Once the ponytail hair is dry, scrunch it to dissolve the gel cast. Then, give your hair a shake: The two textures will look totally different.

WEIGHTING FOR LONGER

How many times has this happened to you? You drive to work while your hair is still wet, and your hair dries up where it has been sitting, right at your shoulders! And all day long you hear, "Oh, you cut your hair!" Or you're about to go out for the evening, but it's humid and your curls have contracted and coiled back like fiddleheads. If you notice this happening to any of your curls as your hair is drying, attach a clip or two at the bottom of each curl until your hair dries. For intense spring-back curls, try attaching the clipped curl strand to your shirt or jacket. (It may sound silly, but it works.) The weight of the clip will stretch out the strand and naturally reduce the spring factor without distorting the curl formation.

Variations on this look:

■ Smooth the top of the hair and pull it into a side ponytail.

■ For a 1920s look, don't pull the ponytail all the way through the holder the third time around, so you have a bun.

■ Place a flower or a hair ornament on the other side of your head.

Pin-Up Curl

This is the "it-looks-complicated-but-it's-not" updo. Simple bobby pins, in all colors and sizes, are anchored, woven, and pinned into the hair.

1 Take the top front section of hair and twist it back to the crown.

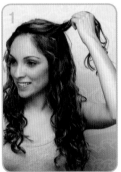
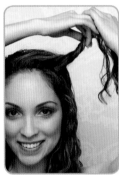

2 Secure the twist to your head either by placing exaggerated amounts of bobby pins for a funky look or using just as many bobby pins as needed along the seam of the twist.

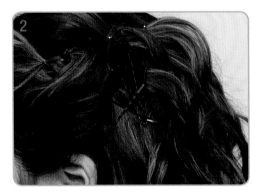

3 Either leave the rest of the hair to flow, or gather it into a low ponytail. Or, the third time you wrap the ponytail holder around your hair, don't pull it all the way through so it looks like a bun.

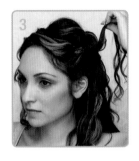

4 For a softer look, gently pry out a few tendrils from around the hairline.

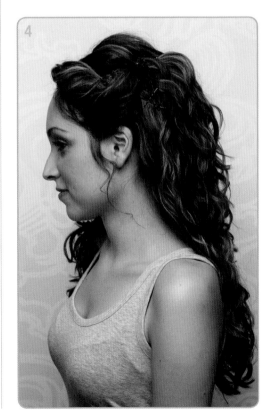

5 If any pieces of hair disperse or frizz during any of these applications, apply a little conditioner and a tiny bit of water, and your hair will return to form.

'20s Revival Wave
WHERE THERE'S A CURL, THERE'S A WAVE

The following method is for curly girls who'd like to be wavy for a day (or more). The process loosens curls without doing any harm to your precious locks. It works best on Botticelli curls with a low frizz factor, but any curly girl can try it. The result is a moist, springy, jazz singer or flapper look.

1 Use the cleansing and conditioning routine described for your curl type. If you have a high frizz factor, leave in some extra conditioner.

2 Step out of the shower and tilt your head to one side. In a downward motion, use a paper towel, microfiber towel, or old cotton T-shirt to pat out excess water. Gently repeat this motion all around your head.

3 While leaning forward with your head tilted in an upside-down position, use your fingers to evenly distribute gel throughout the hair in a downward motion to naturally loosen the curls going from the roots to the ends.

4 Stand upright, and place long clips on the indented concave parts of the wave formations in the hair around the face. If your curls are shrinking violets—they tend to contract when dry—place clips on the ends, which weighs them down to keep length and create a more wavy look.

5 Cover your hair with a hairnet or silk scarf, and allow the hair to air-dry. You can also use a blow-dryer with a diffuser on a low setting, or sit under a hooded dryer.

6 Once the hair is dry, remove the clips, gently shake your hair with your fingers, or allow the hair to stay in its gel cast.

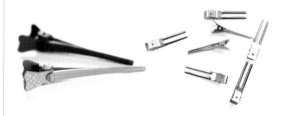

Clips are a curly girl's arsenal. With them, you can lift hair on the crown, make wavy hair curlier, or curly hair wavier, as suggested above.

Love Me Knot

Keeps your hair off of your face by day, and then unravel at night.

1 Grasp the thick section of hair that's hidden near the nape of the neck, under the top layer of hair, and separate it so half is in your right hand and half is in your left.

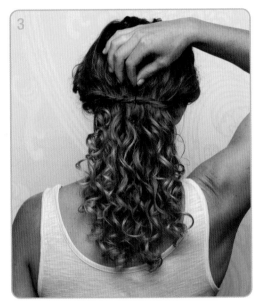

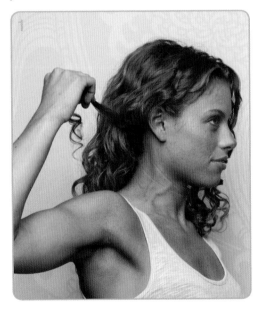

2 Tie the two sections in a knot that wraps around the rest. Loop it three times at the center back of the hair.

3 Use a couple of bobby pins to secure the knot. You can dress up this look with decorative bobby pins or a flower.

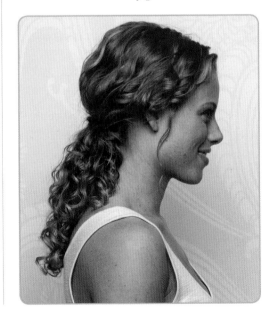

chemo curls

People saw me, not my hair.

I became a hairdresser because I wanted to make people feel great, sexy, and happy about their looks. One of the toughest times is when one of my beloved clients tells me that she has been diagnosed with cancer and is about to undergo chemotherapy. There is not much I can say except that I will be there whenever she needs to see me any time, any place, and anywhere. I remember cutting the hair of a longtime client whose curls were falling out because of chemo. I excused myself for a minute, went to the bathroom, and cried, because I knew how much she had gone through to love and grow the gorgeous curls. Of course, losing her hair was just one hurdle she had to get beyond. I'm so thankful that today she is now cancer free and back with her curls, which look better than ever.

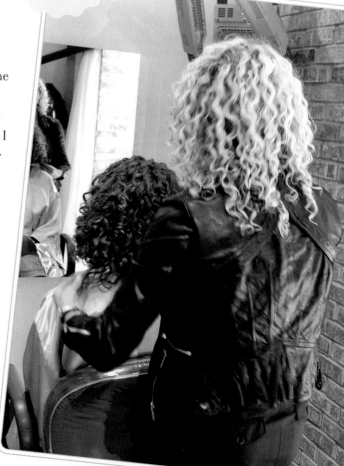

curl confession

Jordan Pacitti *dancer with the Pacific Northwest Ballet*

Going Through It Together

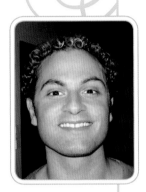

When my partner, Ben (page 175), was going through chemo treatments and his hair began to fall out, I decided to shave my curls off, too. His cancer was a battle we were going to fight together. It felt great emotionally, because I was supporting him (and I loved the way it looked, too). When my hair grew in, my curls were virgin curls again. It made me laugh, seeing my head literally spring curls from the scalp when it grew back. But most of all, I loved supporting my partner through this tough time.

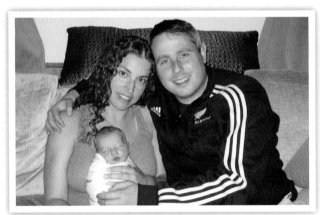

Elizabeth Cantor and family.

Chemo truly cuts through hair and emotions in the most devastating ways. Elizabeth Cantor, a client of mine for more than fifteen years, went through this when she was diagnosed with cancer at the age of thirty-two. "When I was first diagnosed," says Elizabeth, "I thought maybe my hair was strong enough not to fall out from the chemo. It wasn't. Then I had it cut shoulder length, which I thought would make losing it easier. It didn't. It was still traumatic to have it fall out in clumps in the shower. Looking back, I realize that it would have been easier just to have it all shaved off once I was diagnosed so I wouldn't have to go through that. I was bald for six months of my year and a half of treatment. When my hair first started to grow back, it was straight, but then it became curly again. Now, five years later, I'm cancer free and have curls that reach the middle of my back!"

To understand why hair falls out during chemo, I talked with an expert at the American Cancer Society. "Chemotherapy drugs travel throughout the body and attack and damage cells that are reproducing or dividing quickly. Cancer cells do this, but the cells of the hair follicle do this, too, so they're susceptible to the damage of chemo," explains Kimberly Stump-Sutliff, RN, associate medical editor for the American Cancer Society. "Hair loss can be hard to predict. Some patients lose all of their hair, and others do not, even when they take the same drugs." (What's not clear is why formerly straight hair can grow back curly and vice-versa, or why texture and color can change, too.)

After losing their hair, some of my clients wore wigs, but many of them did not. If you do want to wear a wig, you don't have to go straight. Many curly girls donate their hair for wigs for this good cause. And there are many stylish looks besides wigs, like bandannas, hats, berets, and scarves. When the hair starts to grow out, there's nothing more adorable than the pixie haircut. Short, gamine styles like

curl confession

Benjamin Griffiths *dancer with the Pacific Northwest Ballet*

Boy Meets Curls

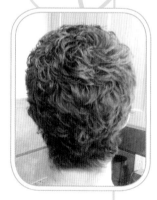

I'd always had thin, stick-straight hair, so when it grew in curly after chemotherapy, I was very surprised. I thought that it would become straight as it thickened and that the curls would be lost with my first trim. But they continued to form. I love the fact that my curly hair has some body, definition, and texture, which add interest and shape that weren't there before. For anyone else who experiences a transition from straight to curly hair after chemo, I say, have fun with it! Take the time to learn to care for your curls. Very few people get to have a drastic change of hair texture in their lifetime, so enjoy experimenting with it. And if you've just been through a grueling battle with cancer, don't fight your curls, too. Instead, love and nurture them!

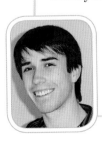

this can make you look younger, springy, and vibrant. Robin Roberts, a co-anchor on *Good Morning America*, wore her hair in a curly pixie style after her cancer treatment, and it looked fabulous.

Once the hair grows in, many women take this opportunity to try something with their color that they might never have done before. A little red, burgundy, or copper highlights throughout can offer a very stylish look, and can help give your complexion a lift since skin may look sallow right after chemo.

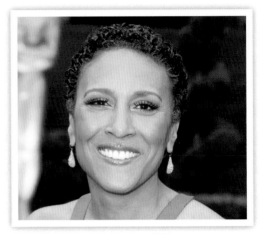

Robin Roberts, co-anchor on GMA

curl confession

Vickie Vela *hairstylist*

A Sister's Legacy of Curls

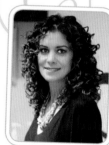

Vickie

My sister, Laura's, hair had always been straight, but grew in curly after she lost it all during cancer treatments. Though she wasn't sure how to manage her new curls, she embraced them and learned to work with them much like she did with cancer. In fact, Laura was one of the rare people who saw this disease as a gift and an opportunity to help others with their struggle and journey.

Laura lost her battle with cancer, but since I am a hairstylist, I have made it my mission as a tribute to my sister to get as many curly girls as I can to embrace their hair—especially the new, postchemo curly girls.

CHEMO CURL TIPS

I asked Elizabeth Cantor for some ideas that could help other women going through chemo, and she offered these tips:

■ If the type of chemo you're having will make your hair fall out, I strongly recommend getting a really, really shorter-than-you-dare haircut. Or if you are brave enough, shave your head completely. As awful as a cancer diagnosis is, the process of your hair falling out is horrifying. I didn't listen to this advice when it was given to me, and the experience was traumatic.

■ Even though you're certain that your hair won't fall out (I thought that only happens to other people), prepare in advance by buying a wig, hats, and bandannas, or decide that you are going to walk around bald. Whatever you choose, make sure that you have something on hand that will make you feel comfortable in public. For cold weather, have some soft hats to cover your head to maintain your body heat.

■ Once I complained to a bald friend of mine that my head looked like a ping-pong ball. He replied, "Well, at least your hair will grow back. I have no choice." He was right! Once your chemo is finished, your hair will start growing back immediately. Within a month after chemo, I retired my wig. I looked like I had a buzz cut, but I didn't care.

■ Formerly curly locks can grow in straight and straight hair can come in curly. It took a couple of months before I had evidence that my curls were going to return.

■ Buy clips, barrettes, and headbands to get through awkward growing-out stages. Find a good stylist who can cut your hair well, so that it grows in nicely. Have fun with each stage, and remember, it's a sign of health when your hair starts to grow back.

curl confession

Noelle Smith *owner, Ellenoire Unique Indulgences*

It's Curl in the Family

L ast year, I got breast cancer and lost my waist-length curls from the chemo. It was hard, but I knew that it was more important to get the right

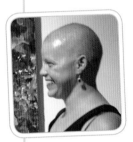

medicine to get rid of the cancer. As my hair grew back, I used a sulfate-free cleanser and botanical conditioner, and took supplements for hair growth, and now my soft, beautiful curls are twice the length of other people's whom I finished chemo with.

Today, I use my store and experience to help women going through chemo and to educate those who have become chemo curly. I think my desire to help others came from my mother, a former hairdresser, who cut everyone's hair in our neighborhood (including my own until I was fourteen). She didn't charge them because her view was that if she could do someone a favor and help out, she would.

When I started selling DevaCurl products in my store, clients kept asking where they could get their hair cut the curly girl way. Frustrated that no one in the area could do it, my mother decided to set up a little place in her house where she could cut hair based on Lorraine's method. Throughout the five years that my mother did this, she had cancer and was going through chemo herself. But even when she didn't feel well, having a client gave her something to get up for. She was passionate about the Curly Girl way of caring for hair. In fact, she cut hair the Curly Girl way until about six weeks before she died.

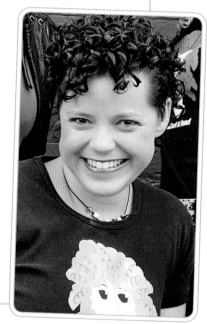

a twelve-step recovery program for curly girls

one curl at a time

Nature versus Nurture. The nature just is and the nurture is you.

It's not enough to admit that you're not straight. The compulsion to abuse products and your precious curly locks is deep-seated and hard to shake. To help curly girls in recovery, we've invented a Twelve-Step Personal Hair Growth and Recovery Program. Since sharing is a necessary part of the program, curly girls are advised to shift their obsession from product abuse to telling others about their curly conversion. When you feel the urge to shampoo, blow-fry, or flat-iron your hair, *stop*, and call a curl-friend sponsor.

The following steps are to be used only as life styling tools. Interpret them in the way that is most helpful to you personally and then follow them as a commitment to yourself. The steps have worked for millions of others who knew they were not naturally straight. They can work for you. In the process of uncovering your curls, you may uncover other parts of yourself long since forgotten.

STEP 1

I admit that I am powerless over my true nature—and that my curly hair will continue to be unmanageable if I deny and abuse it as I have in the past.*

STEP 2

I will stop torturing myself with blow-dryers, brushes, straighteners, rollers, flat irons, and other diabolical ways to straighten my hair, and I will regain my sanity as a curly haired person. I will search my bathroom for such items and throw them away.

You can fight the truth for only so long, but that's not going to make it go away. Make peace now, stop deluding yourself, and see your hair for what it truly is.

STEP 3

I will admit my addiction to going straight and attempt to discover why I have wasted so much of my time in this pursuit. I will accept the nature of my hair and celebrate it rather than fight it.

STEP 4

I will make a decision to turn my curls over to a higher power—the power that created me and my hair—and I will find a curl sponsor to mentor me as a recovering curly girl.

STEP 5

I will give in to the forces of nature, embracing humidity, rain, and wind, facing the elements confidently because I am no longer attempting to go against nature by controlling my curls.

STEP 6

I will make a list of relatives and friends who encouraged my curl denial with compliments about my unnaturally straight hair. I will forgive them as well as the hairdressers who abetted my habit.

STEP 7

I will accept that the scalp and the hair are two different entities with two totally different needs, and I will treat each accordingly.

STEP 8

I will give up shampoo dependency forever and learn how to gently cleanse my curls without turning to products that harm them. No Lather = Soap-briety

STEP 9

I admit that it is my responsibility to take care of my hair in the best way possible. I will learn how to dry it without burning it or harming it, and I will let my curls grow to their full potential.

STEP 10

Whenever I am tempted to go straight, I will call a curl mentor or friend who has embraced her curly destiny and seek her encouragement in living an honest curly life.

STEP 11

I will carry the message by simply being curly to others still living in curl denial.

STEP 12

I will practice these principles that I have learned every day of my life.

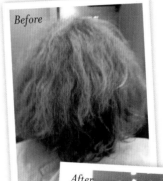

Before

Uncover your buried treasure.

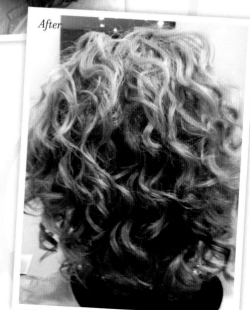

After

astrologi-curls

a curly girl horoscope

capricorn

December 22–January 19

Curls by Virtue, Green by Nature

Capricorn is born in the heart of winter, a product of the longest nights. Capricorns have their own particular vision of the world, so you may at first rebel against your curls. You typically need to be on top; you are determined to overcome all obstacles, and your locks may be one of them. So, let there be curl, reach out to a curl friend, and remember, your hair is on top, not you! To know your curls is to love them.

aquarius

January 20–February 18

Curls R U

Aquarius is the ruler of the hair-waves. As a water sign, you know that curls require the nourishment only a watery environment can provide. You usually confront your hair frustrations well, but if you're slightly insecure, you may demand that your hair change according to your perception of the situation. If you reject your curls, you reject your S-sence. You simply must be true to yourself and your locks. Curl now, or forever hold your hair extensions!

Pisces

February 19–March 20

Obsta-curl Illusions

The days lengthen and thaws begin as Pisces moves beyond herself, always following the movement of the ocean currents and the current trends. You are easily swayed, which is both your strength and your weakness, and this trait also applies to your hair. Sometimes overwhelmed by what's current, you flounder in the face of your curly hair-itage. If you can just ride the wave, you can overcome all obstacles, even if they are illusions.

Aries

March 21–April 19

The Importance of Being Curly

Fiery Aries symbolizes beginnings, the season of renewed life and the start of the sun's annual cy-curl. You are full of fixed ideas, so your boundless curls may threaten you, to the point where you may butt heads with the herd. If you don't rise to the occasion, your hair will! Wear your hair like a well-earned trophy. Surrender. After all, the part of the body ascribed to Aries is the head.

Taurus

April 20–May 20

Ask Not What Your Hair Can Do for You; Ask What You Can Do for Your Hair

Taurus signals the rites of spring, and spring is in the hair. Taurus types who cultivate their gardens may be inclined to get stuck in the mud and might dig in their heels and resist change as a result of many bad hair experiences. Understandable, but don't be closed to new information. Seek a logi-curl approach: You are known to be the goddess of the past. Not figuratively! Be the goddess of the now, and own those natural goddess-given locks.

gemini

May 21–June 21

Love Me, Love My Curls

Gemini brings in the mellow breezes of the summer—and, yes, with it, the humidity. As a twin, staring at your reflection, you have a need for individuality. But you have to accept that going straight and going curly is sway-ving, not committing—and your hair will be neither here nor thair! It's not always a healthy option. You, as the embodiment of the quickening of human intelligence, must accept its truths. Once you get to know your hair's natural grace, you'll accept that every day is a new day.

cancer

June 22–July 22

Better the Curl You Know Than the Curl You Don't

The sun has reached its highest point over the Northern Hemisphere. Open to new ideas, you must nevertheless set limits as a mother must for her adventuresome child. You do not readily accept others, so you may be in need of a worthy curly hairdresser to guide you right. Coexist; it's worthy of you. Then take all your curl knowledge, and pass on the curlove.

Leo

July 23–August 22

You Can Pretend All You Want That You're Not Curly, but That's Not Going to Make the Curls Go Away

At the heat of the high summer, with its intense solar rays, curls are running rampant. It's time to explore your S-sence. Mane-tain what it is you are so fiercely known for. When accepted and loved, your mane will inspire radiance and you will become a leader, encouraging other curly girls to emerge with pride from their dens. If you deny your curls and slink off to try to smooth away the frizzies, by high noon, the untamed will of the frizz will persist.

VIrGO

August 23–September 22

Me, My Curls, and I

At the beginning of the fall harvest, Virgo's humble awareness equips
you early in life with an understanding of your hair's potential.
But with your quest for perfection, you need to remember the old
saying, "It's not perfect, but it's perfect for you." Life is too short to
micromanage one stray curl. Look at the big picture, and stop fussing;
otherwise you'll have big hair. Remember, while your hair is drying,
do not disturb.

LIBra

September 23–October 23

Wear Your Hair, Don't Let It Wear You

This is the fall equinox, when the sun enters the sign of Libra, a h-air
sign that holds an invisible thread connecting us all. Libra rules
relationship, one to one, and you are often one with your hair. If not,
you may pay too much attention to the counsel of others and won't
be in touch with your inner curl. It's like surfing: When you first get
on the surfboard, you may tip from side to side. Only when you are in
balance, will you ride the waves with harmony.

scOrPIO

October 24–November 21

I Really Love You Today

As the nights grow longer, with a suggestion of winter, you
consummate the bond with your hair with intense experimentation.
Together, you must accept and confront its S-sence in pursuit of the
hairy truth. The unbound curl emerges, and it changes hourly, daily,
weekly, monthly, and yearly. Scorpio is attuned to the cy-curl of
death and rebirth, knowing all things in Nature organize themselves
eventually, especially the natural curl!

SAGITTARIUS

November 22–December 21

Curls, Ageless and Evergreen . . .

Born in the winter months, you Sagittarians need your hair to be as carefree and easygoing as you are, as long as you have a logi-curl hair routine to follow. You're the perfect outreach curly girl, since people are always asking you about your curl-ability and you love to tell them!

"There was a little girl
Who had a little curl
Right in the middle of
her forehead.
When she was good
She was very, very good,
But when she was bad,
she was horrid."

—Henry Wadsworth Longfellow

curl it forward

Dear Curly Girl:

You have come to the end of this book, but you may be at the beginning of your curly girl journey. And remember, it is a journey, not a destination, and every day is a new day. I hope that reading the words and stories shared by so many curlies and having a better understanding of your curls' needs, fears, and desires will allow you to be truly free. What I have found—along with many, many of my curly friends—is that this liberating feeling of not fighting against our curls, but rather fighting for them, actually starts to trickle down to other parts of our lives. That's why we feel compelled to share.

The Curly Girl Movement is still very much a grassroots one, beginning with one curly telling another, and curl on, and on. When people constantly stop us and ask, "How do you get your curls to look the way they do?" our boyfriends/partners/ husbands/kids may stand there rolling their eyes, waiting as we pass on our curl know-how to another curly girl waiting to happen. But we know that we have to curl it forward. We have become a culture club unto ourselves. We are all at the beginning, and it's amazing to know that our curly kids may have the opportunity to have a healthy, curly outlook right from the start. Curls are not a trend, they're a lifestyle.

People often tell me, "You've changed my life." But it is you who ultimately changes your life, when you are ready. If anyone may get this little message of curl freedom, it will probably be the curly girl!

Come out, come out wherever you are!
Curl-love forever,

Lorraine

ACKNOWLEDGMENTS

I'd like to start by thanking all the curly girls who are already out there experiencing curl freedom, along with those who are about to discover their buried treasure of curls.

I also want to thank my three children (who, by the way, have never used shampoo) for making me the most grateful curly girl alive. To my son Kaih, who just returned home from five years in the army to be with his wife, Veronica, and daughter, Venaih—thank you and your comrades for all you have done to protect our freedom. To my daughter, Shey, thank you for being my forever muse (even when you didn't want to) and to my son Dylan, who is full of curly ideas, thanks for being my b-roll cameraman (even when you didn't want to).

Many thanks to Michele, who, while writing this book with me, was going through her own curl transformation, growing out her straightened locks to return to her curly hair. Witnessing her newfound love for curls made it worth every single minute. To her daughter, Lily, thank you for all your curly ideas. Thank you, Michele, truly.

Thank you, Carol and Mort Blum, for allowing the use of your apartment, the DevaSpa, and much, much more!

Thanks to David and Jimmy, and to Glenn and Blonde+Co. Thanks to Julio Sandino for outstanding makeup; to Catalina, I'm beyond grateful. To Amy at Tibi and Anni Juan, thank you for the clothes.

To all my curlicious curly girls and guys, whose 100 percent authentic curls grace the pages of *Curly Girl* and its DVD, thank you from the bottom of my heart.

To my business partner, Denis, and all our Devachan–DevaConcepts colleagues, thank you for helping me un-conditionally. My gratitude goes to you always.

Also, a big thanks goes to the amazing Workman gals. They scrunched, trimmed, hyper re-conditioned, and gelled this curly book together. Many thanks to Maisie, Netta, Jenny, Janet, and Lidija, and a special thanks to Anne Kerman and Ruth Sullivan. Ruth, whom I call the T'Ruth, because she is, I am forever grateful for your guidance, input, output, and outlook on nurturing *Curly Girl* right to the end. And last, thank you to Peter Workman (whose hair is completely straight) for listening to David Schiller's idea for *Curly Girl*. Without you, none of this would have taken place in our curly world. Thank you, thank you, thank you, thank you!

Lorraine

Thanks so much to Lorraine, who was both my coauthor and my curly sponsor through the twists and turns of going back to natural curls. Your passion for curls—and life—is awe-inspiring! A million thanks to my parents, Carol and Mort Blum, for always, always being there for me, and to Lily and Jonathan for being the lights of my life—every day I'm grateful that I am your mother. Thanks also to Todd, Vivien, David, Zoe, Melissa, Robyn, and Judy for your constant support, and to my agent, Linda Konner!

Michele

No curls were harmed during the making of this book and DVD.